KV-201-157

PROBLEMS AND POTENTIAL IN INTERNATIONAL HEALTH

MEDWAY CAMPUS LIBRARY

This book is due for re   date stamped
          but may be r
          Fines wi

WITHDRAWN
FROM
UNIVERSITIES
AT
MEDWAY
LIBRARY

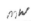

Problems and Potential in International Health
Transdisciplinary Perspectives

Pieter Streefland (editor)

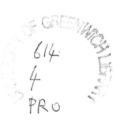

614
4
PRO

KIT Press
1998

Problems and Potential in International Health is co-published
by the Royal Tropical Institute and Het Spinhuis Publishers

ISBN 90 6832 120 X
[KIT-Press edition, available in the rest of the world]

ISBN 90 5589 116 9
[Het Spinhuis Publishers edition, available in The Netherlands]

© 1998 The authors

No part of this publication may be recorded or transmitted in any form or by any
means, electronic or mechanical, including photocopy, recording, or any information
storage and retrieval system, without permission of the copyright owner.

Cover design: Jos Hendrix
Lay-out: Hanneke Kossen
Production: Het Spinhuis Publishers
Printed and bound in the Netherlands

Royal Tropical Institute | KIT-Press
P.O. Box 95001, 1090 HA Amsterdam, The Netherlands
Telephone: 31 - 20 - 56 88 277, fax: 31 - 20 - 56 88 286
e-mail: kitpress@kit.nl, website: www.kit.nl

Contents

Acknowledgements

The editor wishes to thank the directors of the Royal Tropical Institute for their support in organizing the series of lectures from which the essays originate and for enabling him to prepare this volume. He also gratefully acknowledges the financial support from the Fund for Development Related Activities of the University of Amsterdam.

Introduction:
Problems and Potential in International Health

One thing is clear, the concept international health, and the fields of science and action it denotes, concern change: change in health, health care and disease control as defined and highlighted from different disciplinary perspectives. A prime example is the staggering drop in infant and child mortality, with the concomitant increase in life expectation, which began worldwide earlier this century and pushed through several plateaus after the second world war, particularly in the developing countries. A health social scientist or public health specialist would point out that this global change in mortality reflects a general improvement in living conditions. From an epidemiological perspective, though, it can also be seen as the result of changes in the prevalence of certain, particularly infectious, diseases. Some diseases like smallpox have disappeared, while others like malaria are now limited to specific regions. From yet another perspective, the changes can be ascribed to the development and widespread use of new medical technologies, e.g. vaccination.

To consider the larger scale and the patterning of these changes in morbidity and mortality, the concept of transition has been introduced. If the perspective taken is narrow, stressing shifts from infectious disease to chronic disease prevalence, or wide, adding changes in behaviour patterns and other health determinants to this, authors use the term epidemiological or health transition, respectively (Omran 1971; Caldwell 1990; Frenk et al. 1994).

We must be careful when using such general notions of international health, because they easily conceal another major characteristic, namely that of heterogeneity. International health, in the sense of a global condition stands for differentiation, sometimes even polarization, in disease and mortality patterns, between regions, social and economic classes, ethnic groups, men and women. Thus, international health can be addressed in the widest, global sense, and also in a more restricted sense, studying problems or conditions pertaining to a specific contradiction or differential pattern. This is most evident when regarding health and health care in developing countries, as done by a number of the present essays. In this introduction I largely write about international health in this more restricted sense, focusing on developing countries.

Again, different perspectives may be the point of departure for description and understanding of differentiation. Epidemiologists may emphasize the change in habitat of certain vectors as a result of public health measures and changing agricultural practices. More economically oriented health social scientists may point to differential access to resources as the explanation of part of the variation in mortality and morbidity. Some medical anthropologists, on the other hand, may discuss the issues in terms of changing cultural identities and practices, rooted in relations of domination.

This brings us to a third aspect of international health, namely the perspectives from which it is approached as a subject of research. Changes have been brought about by disciplinary development and rapprochement. The emergence of tropical medicine as a specialty at the end of the last century may be seen as a watershed in this respect (Worboys 1976). (Sub)disciplines such as tropical epidemiology, medical anthropology, health economics, have matured, each studying issues of international health from their own epistemological assumptions, using different paradigms and methods to create knowledge and phrasing that knowledge in their own discursive language. A new development has been that scientists from distinctive (sub-) disciplines have increasingly tried to overcome prejudice and misunderstanding, in order to obtain a more holistic view of the developments in international health.

International health as a field of study implies action-related or applied research into health and health care problems for a range of particular biomedical disciplines. One example is the intertwining of tropical medicine and public health, usually termed tropical hygiene. In the social sciences this strong inclination to apply the results of research to action and to choose one's aims and subjects for research accordingly is far weaker. There are, in contrast, many health social scientists who emphasize a more reflective and critical role for their discipline. This dual emphasis has been conceptually translated as anthropology *in* (applied) and anthropology *of* (reflective) medicine.

The growth of an international health policy, including collective action by national states and the formulation of international rules, provides the fourth perspective. In the nineteenth century this concerned particularly an initiative of the colonial powers with the principal aim to curtail the spread of epidemics. Since the Second World War, with its aftermath of decolonization, it has become a much more global effort to enhance public health and control disease, involving international agencies like the World Bank, UNICEF and the World Health Organization, national states, and non-government organizations. The agendas constantly change their emphasis as new policies enter the limelight, stressing the health problems of another group or new ways to tackle such problems.

In a way, this internationalization of health policy, together with the global significance of certain diseases – epidemics are not concerned with national borders – may be seen as the representation of the process of globalization in the field of health. But this is only part of the story. There are significant elements of the process of globalization which are crucial to developments in international health and demand study. First, there is the increased movement of people and goods, which is, e.g., instrumental in the spreading of infectious disease. Second, the proliferation of medical technology, both simple and sophisticated, to all corners of the earth is leading to lower mortality. Third, the meanings people attach to such technology also circumnavigate the globe and affect their actual use. Finally, increased global communication between those involved in the study of international health or in the practical pursuit of health improvement provides shortcuts to better understanding, prevention and cure.

Problems and potential in international health

Not surprisingly, the multifaceted concept international health also harbours a wide array of problems, a number of which are considered in the following essays. There are constantly fluctuating global patterns of contracting – sometimes even disappearing (e.g. smallpox and possibly shortly polio) – or expanding and (re)emerging disease. These last two categories form the major problem. We are faced with old infectious diseases, such as malaria and tuberculosis, which are, in fact, out of control. But there is also the increasingly important rise in chronic diseases and disabilities, which cross geographic and socio-economic borders (Murray & Lopez 1996). AIDS is still the foremost emerging disease, while most of the 'smaller plagues', like Ebola and Lassa fever, have fortunately remained so. One more category should be added, that of the forgotten diseases, like occupational diseases in most developing countries. Undernutrition and related morbidity among women is another example (see Kusin, this volume). Sometimes a cluster of forgotten afflictions suddenly becomes the focus of attention, as has been recently the case with reproduction-related disorders.

Another range of problems concerns health care and disease control: our overall capacity of coping with health problems. This involves both the technical domain of the lack of effective therapies and preventive interventions, as in the case of malaria and AIDS, and the inefficiency and ineffectiveness of health services accompanied by the low morale of health professionals. These latter problems, sometimes indicated as contraction of the services (Streefland et al. 1995), have made deep inroads into the relation between the public and the private health care sectors under certain conditions. Problems of national coping capacity include the willingness of political elites in developing countries to allot sufficient budget to a public health department, and the need for a rich country's government to set aside funds in time to deal with the potential disease burden associated with an increasingly elderly population. It also includes the consequences of destruction of infrastructure in the course of national violence and breakdown of states.

A third set of problems may be described as the lack of coping capacity among the afflicted. These are the problems faced by the ill and their caretakers, for instance when they are dealing with the health services, usually called problems of access and affordability. There are also the implications of using medical technology, including drugs, under conditions of different interpretative rationalities than those who designed the technologies and those who promote them in the health services and the market.

Finally, I want to mention problems associated with research, to understand the causes of disease and the ways in which it spreads, to find new technologies, to test interventions, to implement the interventions, to comprehend how users perceive new technologies and apply them. In all these areas we are faced with problems of developing new concepts and paradigms, inventing new methodologies to obtain valid data, learning new ways to transcend the disciplinary borders and pitfalls, and understanding how to apply our knowledge most easily, harmlessly and cheaply to improve health.

There is also a positive side to international health. Some developments do exist which counter or mitigate the problems just mentioned, although finding them is harder work than defining the problems. I shall list a few, namely those most relevant to the following essays. The most important ones are social and economic improvements. Although there is still appalling poverty in many societies, the increase in poverty, which has long been obvious, appears to be relenting in some developing countries such as Bangladesh and Mali. In addition, literacy and numeracy are on the increase, primarily among the most deprived, namely women. Yet, we cannot speak of a general positive change in poverty conditions which have been and are such a determining force behind health development and its absence.

Nent of new medicaext, it is developml technology (including the acceptance of traditional resources like herbal drugs) is taking us further. However, medical technology is not always beneficial, nor necessary, nor reaching those most in need. But it is, undeniably, a major way to control a major problem: expanding and emerging disease.

A third promising aspect is that there is innovative capacity in health policy. First, this includes uncovering groups and social categories who have lagged behind in terms of access and attention for their problems, women being the prime, but not only, example. Second, this capacity covers setting new priorities and choosing new principles, as in the case of primary health care. Third, it entails the resolve to come to terms with devastating problems as in the case of health reform policies now prevailing in several African countries. Fourth, it is embedded in a large number of social networks with a global span and a number of closely related international organizations. Again, we need to be cautious: the policy innovation is not infrequently of a small scale or for a short duration, and seldom do the organizations involved work closely together.

Lastly, the rapprochement between different scientific disciplines offers an important, exciting and promising development. We observe, as in this volume, anthropologists and sociologists who approach their problems using epidemiological knowledge and medical professionals who are aware of the social and economic determinants of health and realize the importance of understanding the interpretations which patients attach to their health problems. However, there is still some distance to go before it becomes self-evident and for medical and social scientists to define and approach problems jointly, learning from each other and relying upon each other, supported by facilitating institutions.

The chapters

The present volume originated from an initiative in disciplinary rapprochement. In early 1997 I organized a series of lectures by social and medical scientists working at two institutions in Amsterdam, the Royal Tropical Institute and the University of Amsterdam. Both these institutions have a long tradition in the study of health problems in developing countries, which started in the first quarter of this century with the subject of tropical hygiene and the training of medical doctors who were going to work in the then Netherlands Indies. I invited both a medical professional and a sociologist or anthropologist to present their views on six broad topics. The 11 essays – due to illness one presentation could not be given – presented here are based on these lectures. Their sequence reflects the original pairing, though a few changes have been made. Obviously, the discursive style of the individual chapters varies and reflects the disciplinary background, working experience and interests of their authors.

The initial four chapters, written by a tropical medicine specialist and three social scientists, all concern epidemics. In Chapter 1 Kager discusses the new epidemics, such as Ebola and Lassa fever, about which we currently hear and read so much. He clarifies the conceptual intricacies related to the use of terms like (re)emerging infections, and locates the new epidemics in the landscape of global health. He emphasizes the importance of old, persisting infectious diseases, like African trypanosomiasis. He concludes with a review of prevention and control of new epidemics.

De Swaan, in Chapter II, examines under what conditions rich countries would collectively and decisively seek to ameliorate public heaıılth facilities in poor countries. His starting point is the nineteenth century cholera epidemics in Europe and the ensuing improvements in European urban sanitation. He describes how this occurred through a process of collective action to produce the new public goods of sanitation and drinking water supply. Subsequently, he discusses how a similar process of collective action toward public health improvements in the South could be rooted in contemporary global epidemic interdependencies.

Since usually little is known about the social effects of epidemics until afterwards, Streefland endeavours in Chapter III to find directions for the prospective social science research required to fill this gap. He reviews how past plague and cholera epidemics have led to specific forms of temporary and long-term social change. To clarify the social science perspective on epidemics, he then distinguishes biomedically defined epidemics from imagined epidemics and social epidemics. He concludes by listing basic research questions on which studies of the social consequences of contemporary epidemics could focus.

Varkevisser, in Chapter IV, discusses innovation in social science methodology in research on HIV/AIDS transmission and control. Drawing on her broad experience in Southern Africa in general and, more specifically, Tanzania she highlights participatory methodologies and the required collaboration between epidemiologists and social scientists. She further discusses new approaches in the study of sexual relations and practices, and of gender inequality in sexual relations.

The next three chapters, by two public health physicians and a social scientist, focus on specific aspects of changing health care in developing countries.

In Chapter V Kusin discusses the Safe Motherhood Initiative (SMI) from a medical perspective, with a focus on non-infectious morbidity of women of reproductive age. Drawing on her research on the undernutrition of women in Indonesia, she shows the importance of their chronic energy deficiency, exacerbated by nutritional stress surrounding birth and lactation, as a major factor causing problems related to reproduction. Subsequently, when discussing policy matters she criticizes the lack of nutritional elements in the SMI, emphasizes the need for participatory priority setting, and highlights the importance of attention for adolescents as a beginning for safe motherhood and of income-generating programmes for women as a sound fundament for improvement in livelihood.

Hardon, in Chapter VI, looks into reproductive health problems in the South from a medical anthropological perspective. Presenting results from studies on fertility regulation in Asia and Africa, she shows how empirical data can be instrumental in finding appropriate and effective interventions. She relates poor Philippine urban women's views and use of the contraceptive pill to their living conditions and requirements. Understanding how Mozambiquan women cope with the problem of fertility in their specific socio-economic and cultural context provides a sound basis for formulating gender and culture-sensitive interventions.

Chabot, in Chapter VII, describes and contrasts changes in public health care in two African countries, Zambia and Guinee Bissau, on the basis of his personal involvement. In Zambia the health reforms which are presently being implemented are far-reaching and have strong political undertones. In Guinee Bissau a more restricted and rather technically aligned programme to change the health sector is underway. Both forms of change will lead to improvements, though there are many difficulties ahead, such as appropriately combining equity and efficiency.

One of the intriguing problems in technology development is how to overcome the gap between the research environment and the practical application. The next two chapters, by a sociologist and two medical scientists, are devoted to this issue.

Blume, in Chapter VIII, gives a critical assessment of a number of steps on the road from 'bench to bush' in development of new technologies, using the case of vaccine development. He discusses important concepts like safety and efficacy and shows how their meanings differ in different situations. He also reviews some essential aspects of data collection during clinical trials. He looks into the role of global alignments like the Children's Vaccine Initiative, and examines the position of the pharmaceutical industry in regard to vaccine technology.

In Chapter IX Terpstra and Smits describe the different steps in the development of a diagnostic test for *leptospirosis*. This test has been developed at a biomedical research laboratory in Amsterdam but needs to be used in the South. He also discusses the difficulties the laboratory has to face when, in addition to research, it needs to become oriented towards production and marketing of the new technology.

Finally, a pharmacologist and an anthropologist examine questions about medicines and the way they are used.

In Chapter X Van der Geest discusses the use and misuse of pharmaceuticals in the South. He notes that pharmaceuticals are extremely popular and widely available. Usually, sick people use medicines as a form of self-medication. He continues to discuss three cultural processes which guide their perceptions and behaviour: commoditization, cultural reinterpretation and symbolization. He also discusses the important subject of different rationalities in drug use, by focusing on the rationality of inappropriate drug use. He concludes with remarks on counteracting the misuse of drugs.

Van Wilgenburg, in Chapter XI, reviews the important contribution of herbal medicines to global health. Using the case of anti-malarials and anti-cancer drugs, he shows how plants are and can be sources of medicines. He demonstrates the potential of ethnobotany to find promising leads for new drugs, and discusses ethical problems that arise when herbal resources in developing countries are used by pharmaceutical companies from the North. He pleads for strengthening the control of herbal medicine production by Southern organizations and governments.

Literature

Caldwell, J.C.

1990 'Introductory thoughts on health transition.' In: J.C. Caldwell, S. Findley, P. Caldwell, G. Santow, W. Cosford, J. Braid & D. Broers-Freeman, *What we know about the health transition: the cultural, social and behavioural determinants of health*. Health transition series, Vol. 1, No. 2. Canberra: Health Transition Centre, Australian National University.

Frenk, J., J. Bobadilla, C. Stern, T. Frejka & R. Lozano

1994 'Elements for a theory of the health transition'. In: L.C. Chen, A. Kleinman & N.C. Ware (eds), *Health and social change in international perspective*. Boston: Harvard School of Public Health, pp. 25-51.

Murray, J.L. & A.D. Lopez (eds)

1996 *The global burden of disease. A comprehensive assessment of mortality and disability from diseases, injuries, and risk factors in 1990 and projected to 2020*. Cambridge: Harvard School of Public Health.

Omran, A.R.

1971 'The epidemiologic transition: A theory of the epidemiology of population change.' *Milbank memorial fund quarterly* 49: 509-538.

Streefland, P.H., J.W. Harnmeijer & J. Chabot

1995 'Implications of economic crisis and structural adjustment policies for PHC in the periphery.' In: J. Chabot, J.W. Harnmeijer & P.H. Streefland (eds), *African primary health care in times of economic turbulence*. Amsterdam: KIT Press, pp. 11-19.

Worboys, M.

1976 'The emergence of tropical medicine: A study in the establishment of a scientific specialty.' In: G. Lemaine, R. Macleod, M. Mulkay & P. Weingart (eds), *Perspectives on the emergence of scientific disciplines*. Paris: Mouton, pp. 75-89.

CHAPTER I

New Epidemics:
Possibilities for Prevention and Control

PIET A. KAGER

Infectious diseases are back in the public limelight. They are discussed in the lay and professional press, on radio and television. We are given the impression that new and well-known infectious diseases are menacing us, with catastrophies threatening imminently. We hear about new epidemics, killer viruses, flesh-eating bacteria, deadly bugs, resistant bacteria, emerging and re-emerging diseases. A new journal *Emerging Infectious Diseases* appeared, the first conference on Emerging Infections took place (Boston, 11-13 June 1997). Infectious diseases are in fashion.

The novel *The Hot Zone* by Richard M. Preston (1994) about an Ebola outbreak became a bestseller. In 1995 the film *Outbreak*, about an Ebola-like virus was released. The book *The Coming Plague* by the science journalist Laurie Garrett (1995) is a thorough, extensively referenced description of new diseases and their causal agents and of old agents in new clothes. Garrett discusses these new and well-known diseases in the context of changes in public health and society, against a background of declining interest in communicable diseases, reduced budgets and less priority for education in the field of infectious diseases. She discusses the new challenges in relation to politics and bureaucracy and concludes that the situation is far from ideal.

We saw panic about plague in India and reactions out of proportion to the scale and threat of the outbreak (see also Streefland, this volume). India suffered large economic losses because of the unreasonable reactions of trading companies, air and shipping companies, airport and harbour authorities. Travellers cancelled trips without compensation, at least in The Netherlands where the authorities did not advise against travelling to India. In contrast, an epidemic increase of dengue in and around New Delhi in 1996 did not cause any unrest among travellers although the risk of catching dengue, and probably even of catching the complicated form of the disease with shock, bleeding tendency, and death, was much higher than the risk of catching plague, or even getting near to a plague victim.

The enormous publicity surrounding the Ebola epidemic in Kikwit, Zaire, in 1995, with a few hundred deaths, was completely out of proportion to the few lines on a meningitis outbreak that raged in Nigeria at the same time, killing thousands. The smaller outbreaks of Ebola in 1996 in Gabon were no longer newsworthy.

Cholera in Latin America, a new cholera strain (*Vibrio cholerae* O139) with the potential of initiating a new worldwide epidemic (a pandemic), a new hanta virus causing a severe lung disease (hantavirus pulmonary syndrome), mad cow disease (bovine spongiform encephalopathy, BSE), the hamburger or beefburger diarrhoea syndrome due to *Escherichia coli* O157: H7, all hit the headlines.

Are we indeed threatened by new and well-known infections, are we in danger? Or have we forgotten about epidemics, thinking that infectious diseases had been conquered? Is the panic caused by ignorance? Are we witnessing new epidemics and, if so, what is new about them? Are epidemics getting out of control? Do we need new ways and means of prevention and control? Are we sufficiently equipped for the new challenges, if they exist at all?

After a brief introduction to the definitions of epidemics, emerging and re-emerging diseases, in this contribution some well-known and some new infections are discussed. These diseases are put in the perspective of the globally important causes of disease and death. A historical perspective on epidemics is explored, and their causes and ways of prevention and control described.

Infectious diseases in the context of global morbidity and mortality

What do we mean when we talk about epidemics, about emerging and re-emerging diseases? Benenson (1990) defines epidemics as: 'the occurrence in a community or region of cases of an illness (or an outbreak) clearly in excess of expectancy'. The number of cases is relative to the agent, to the size and type of population, to previous exposure, and to time and place of occurrence. Epidemics are not necessarily about huge numbers of victims. Some infectious agents are highly contagious and infect many people in a short period of time (influenza), others spread much less easily (tuberculosis).

A few cases of diphtheria in The Netherlands now would be an epidemic, because there has been no diphtheria for many years, mainly due to the high vaccination coverage. What is 'epidemic' in one part of the world may be 'normal' (expected) elsewhere. In the 1960s a hundred or more cases of smallpox were normal in Ethiopia or India (not in The Netherlands); in the 1980s two cases of smallpox in Ethiopia, after the eradication of this disease, would have been epidemic and a cause for great concern.

Let us be clear that epidemics are not only about infectious diseases. They are about any condition, also about chemical intoxication, injury, road accidents, drug addiction, smoking-related disorders, shell fish poisoning and so on.[1]

In this contribution the emphasis is on infectious diseases, but we should note that 2/3 of the death toll worldwide is due to non-infectious diseases and conditions. In the *World Health Report 1996* the World Health Organization (WHO) paid a lot of attention to infectious diseases. WHO estimated that in 1995, 51.9 million people died worldwide, of these 17.3 million (33%) due to infectious diseases, 11 million of whom were children below 5 years of age (WHO 1996a). The *World Health Report 1997* was more concerned about non-infectious, chronic conditions. It mentioned that of the estimated 52 million deaths in 1996, 40 million were in the developing countries, of these 17 million (43.0%) were due to infectious and parasitic diseases, about 10 million (24.5%) due to circulatory diseases, 4 million (9.5%) due to cancers and 2 million (4.8%) due to non-infectious respiratory diseases.

Infectious and parasitic diseases remain the most important killer conditions in developing countries, especially among the most disadvantaged, but chronic diseases also emerge as major causes of death and disability there, accounting for almost 40% of all deaths (WHO 1997a).[2]

When focussing on infectious diseases, we should realize that the big killers among them still are respiratory infections and diarrhoeal diseases in children (Table 1). Of all infections due to a single pathogen, tuberculosis is still the leader, claiming about 3 million lives per year. Preventable infections like hepatitis B, measles, tetanus and whooping cough are important causes of death, followed at a distance by parasitic infections like leishmaniasis or worms.

Common, indeed daily infectious problems and the susceptibility of infectious organisms to drugs that people can afford are much more significant and have a much greater bearing on health, morbidity and mortality than the much more 'fashionable' infections of Ebola and Sin Nombre virus. A good example of a widescale, very worrisome problem is that

H. influenzae and *S. pneumoniae*, the pneumococcus, are becoming more and more resistant to the commonly used and cheap antibiotics, also in the tropics. Thus, we are losing some of the most useful and affordable antibiotics as a means of controlling the two bacteria that are the major causes of death in children.

Table 1 Major infectious diseases causing death. 1995 estimates

	$\times 10^6$
acute lower resp. infection *(not measles, pertussis, HIV)*	4.4
diarrhoea *(not measles, HIV)*	3.1
tuberculosis	3.1
malaria	2.1
hepatitis B	1.1
measles	1.1
AIDS	1.1
neonatal tetanus	0.5
whooping cough	0.4
leishmaniasis	0.08

On definitions

With a focus on infectious diseases, in particular new epidemics, the question arises 'what is new, what is old'? Since 1973, 30 new pathogens and diseases have been identified. Table 2 shows a selection of 12 new agents. Prominent in this list are viruses: Ebola, Hantaan and human immunodeficiency virus (HIV), two viruses related to leukaemia/lymphoma, two hepatitis viruses and two other viruses causing haemorrhagic fever.

Because of space constraints I will not discuss food- and water-borne epidemics.[3] HIV infection is certainly extremely important and new but is discussed regularly elsewhere and will not be dealt with here.

The concepts *emerging* and *re-emerging* infections are often used nowadays. They are also applied to well-known foes like cholera, meningococcal meningitis and salmonellosis (WHO 1996a). The terms are usually somewhat loosely defined.

The editorial policy of the journal *Emerging Infectious Diseases* (Anonymous 1996) states:

Emerging infections are new or newly identified pathogens or syndromes recognized in the past two decades. Re-emerging infections are known pathogens or syndromes that are increasing in incidence, expanding into new geographic areas, affecting new populations, or threatening to increase in the near future.

The WHO (1996a: 15) calls emerging infectious diseases:

those whose incidence in humans has increased during the last two decades or which threatens to increase in the near future. The term also refers to newly appearing infectious diseases, or diseases that are spreading to new geographical areas. It also refers to diseases that were easily controlled by chemotherapy and antibiotics, but which have developed antimicrobial resistance.

Table 2 Aetiological agents of 12 selected diseases, first recognized since 1976

1976	*Cryptosporidium parvum*
1977	Ebola virus
1977	Hantaan virus
1980	Human T-lymphotropic virus 1
1982	Escherichia coli O157: H7
1982	Human T-lymphotropic virus 2
1983	Human immunodeficiency virus
1988	Hepatitis E virus
1989	Hepatitis C virus
1991	Guanarito virus
1992	Vibrio cholerae O139
1994	Sabia virus

Louria (1996: 59) defines emerging infections as those that are either newly described or, alternatively, are known but appear in new geographic areas or increase markedly in frequency, particularly in compromised hosts. Re-emerging infections are previously well described and either occur in new geographic areas or reappear in the same geographic area after a period of relative or complete dormancy.

But what exactly is meant by the two decades in the first two definitions and what Louria feels is 'newly described' are not clear. Is it two decades from a particular year, or is it looking back from the year of writing? Cryptosporidium was recognized in 1976. Is it from 1997 onwards no longer an emerging infection? Can we in 1997 still call it 'newly described'? Probably new pathogens discovered from 1976 onwards are meant. Similarly, the definition of re-emerging is not really satisfactory, as it is so broad that it may accommodate any pathogen.

Appropriate working definitions, based on the previous ones, would probably be: *(re-) emerging* infectious diseases are those whose incidence in humans has increased since 1976 or those that threaten to increase in the near future. They include:

a   newly appearing infectious diseases;
b   diseases that are spreading to new geographic areas;
c   diseases caused by pathogens with new pathogenicity;
d   diseases that were formerly controlled by antibiotics but have developed antimicrobial resistance.

This approach leads to a wide range of agents and diseases and may in the end encompass all infections. In one issue of the journal *Emerging Infectious Diseases* (1996, vol 2, no 3) one finds, for example, the following range of diseases:

– *Haemophilus influenzae* infection;
– microsporidiosis;
– coccidioidomycosis;
– HIV infection;
– morbillivirus infection in dolphins;
– rickettsiosis;
– legionella like amoeba infection;
– enterovirus 71 infection;
– bancroftian filariasis;
– yellow fever in Kenya;
– paramyxovirus infection in bats;
– *Mycobacterium genavensis* infection; and
– equine morbillivirus infection.

This list includes well-known, very familiar and common pathogens like *H. influenzae*, but also new ones like morbillivirus in dolphins and equine morbillivirus in man which very recently occurred in Australia. Bancroftian filariasis, a chronic, well-known condition, debilitating but not normally fatal, is in the list because of its increase in the Nile Delta. This increase was probably related to the construction of the Aswan Dam.

A neglected (re-)emerging infectious disease: Sleeping sickness (African trypanosomiasis)

The change from worse to better to worse in Zaire

Malaria receives much attention as an (re-) emerging disease, while African trypanosomiasis, sleeping sickness, seems to be neglected.[4] Trypanosomiasis is an old scourge that devastated large parts of Africa in the early years of this century. In the following decennia, the situation improved considerably.

In 1906 Winston Churchill declared in the House of Commons that the population of Uganda had been reduced from 6.5 million to 2.5 million due to trypanosomiasis (Ekwanzala et al. 1996: 1427). By the late 1950s the number of cases had dropped drastically.

In Zaire reliable data are available from 1926. In 1930 there were 33,562 new cases in Zaire, but by the end of the 1950s there were 'only' about 1,000 new cases per year. This reduction was almost exclusively due to the introduction of a health infrastructure with mobile teams, active and passive case finding and treatment.

Zaire became independent in 1960 and civil war broke out and raged through the country until 1967. In the 1970s about 5,000 new cases were seen per year. By 1989 this had increased to 10,000 due to national mismanagement and the deteriorating socio-economic situation. From the early 1990s the socio-economic decline accelerated rapidly with, in some years, hyperinflation of 100,000%, the local money became useless, and a barter economy developed in many rural parts. Communications were extremely difficult, public health facilities were not functioning, and only mission hospitals continued their services.

The control of trypanosomiasis relied on mobile teams, which in turn depended on foreign aid that was withdrawn for several years because of the human rights situation in the country and the lack of democratic, political and economic reform. Aid was to some extent resumed in 1993. In 1994, 19,340 new cases were found in those parts of the endemic area where the teams could enter. The situation is such that now mortality due to trypanosomiasis equals that due to AIDS. The number of deaths due to trypanosomiasis in 1994 was at least 80 times that due to Ebola fever in Kikwit in 1995 (Ekwanzala et al. 1996), but did we ever hear about this in the media?

Why could this tremendous increase in incidence of sleeping sickness occur? As so often the case, it is a question of politics and money. Under the dictatorship of Mobutu, the country and its infrastructure, including the medical infrastructure, were ruined. Salaries were not paid, there were no means or materials, no drugs for treatment or prevention. This neglect of the medical infrastructure was shown to the world during the Ebola outbreak in Kikwit (see below).

I discuss the case of trypanosomiasis at some length because it so clearly demonstrates the problems with which we are confronted. Much is known about the parasite, about the disease, about the epidemiology. We know so much about possibilities of control that there has been success in several areas. Yet dramatic situations like the one in Zaire do occur.

Despite available means, no prevention and control

The disease is especially prevalent in the Western part of the country where the West African type of trypanosomiasis prevails, with a relatively simple transmission: man – tsetse-fly – man. In the eastern part of the country small pockets of East African trypanosomiasis are found. There the situation is more complicated because of the existence of a reservoir in wild animals. Thus, case finding and treatment become necessary, but the reservoir of disease remains untouched. Large-scale fly traps are part of a solution; a vaccine would also help.

To break the transmission cycle in West Africa, one can do something about the fly (insecticides, traps, genetic manipulation, sterile males) or about man (case finding and treatment). There is no vaccine and no protective medicine.

For the treatment of the early stage, we have pentamidine and suramin, acceptable drugs although far from ideal. They have to be injected intravenously or intramuscularly several times and are relatively toxic. For late stage disease with involvement of the central nervous system, there is an old arsenical drug. The drug is toxic and kills at least 5% of all those who take it.

There is an alternative drug, eflornithine, which is effective for West African trypanosomiasis, even in very late stage disease. It was called the 'resurrection drug', a 'miracle drug'. Also this drug is far from ideal because it has to be given intravenously several times per day, which is cumbersome, increases costs and is only possible in clinics with some means and personnel. Eflornithine is much less toxic than arsenicals, but unfortunately it is expensive, so expensive that no country with endemic sleeping sickness can afford it. Thus, there is no regular commercial demand, and the producer of eflornithine is not interested in production. Because of pressure from the environmental movement and a low profit margin, the producer of the arsenical wants to stop production. At the request of the WHO, both producers still produce, and the WHO distributes, but it is uncertain how long this can go on. The WHO is trying to get eflornithine manufactured somewhere else, e.g. in India or Egypt, but has not been successful so far.

This is the situation: a well-known epidemic with new dimensions. Our knowledge about possibilities for prevention and control is satisfactory, we have reasonable tools. It has been shown that trypanosomiasis could be controlled to the extent that it would not be a threat to public health anymore. Yet trypanosomiasis is back as a serious public health problem.

The animal connection

Many new infections are *zoonoses*, diseases with an animal reservoir. They emerge in man after environmental change, often a man-made one, or due to changes in climatic conditions. I briefly discuss a number of the new zoonotic diseases, listed in Table 3.

Table 3 Zoonoses that appeared in man in relation to ecological disruption

country	virus	known since	site	activity
Argentina	Junin	1940-	maize fields	harvest
Bolivia	Machupo	1952	villages	unknown
Venezuela	Guanarito	1989	forest	clearing
Brazil	Sabia	1990	countryside	unknown
China Korea Balkans	Hantaan	< 1000 1951-1953	countryside/ forest	work in bushes/ forest
Scandinavia W-Europe	Puumala	since 1950-s	countryside/ forest	work in forest, barns, sheds
USA (S.America)	Sin Nombre and others	1993	countryside	camping; work; unknown

Modifications in agricultural practices in the maize-growing pampas of Argentina in the 1940s caused changes in the rodent population that carries the Junin virus. During harvesting agricultural workers came into contact with the rodents and their excrement and acquired Argentinian haemorrhagic fever. Nowadays, those especially at risk are the operators of combines as they suspend clouds of infective dust and create aerosols of infected blood when they crush animals. The virus was identified in 1958, a vaccine was developed and a vaccination campaign is now taking place in Argentina.

In 1952 Machupo, also harbouring in mice, caused an epidemic of haemorrhagic fever in a village in Bolivia; it came back in 1974. It is not clear how and why.

Guanarito appeared in Venezuela in 1989 when people cleared an area in a forest and stirred up dust contaminated with dried rat urine and excrement with virus.

In 1990 in Sao Paulo an agricultural engineer died of Sabia, an arenavirus of rodents. Initially, he was diagnosed as suffering from yellow fever. A worker in a laboratory in the USA where specimens of the victim had been sent became infected 4 years later. He survived.

Haemorrhagic fever with a renal syndrome, now known to be caused by a hanta virus residing in rodents, was mentioned in ancient Chinese literature more than 1,000 years ago. In the Korean war the UN troops suffered extensively from this disease. The virus circulates in large areas of China, Korea, Russia and in the Balkans.

In Scandinavia and Western Europe a similar but milder disease, *nephropathia epidemica*, is known. It is caused by the *Puumala* virus, with a reservoir in the bank vole and other mice. Infection is transmitted by inhalation of dust while working in the forest, in barns and sheds in the countryside (Garrett 1995; Le Guenno 1995).

One of the newer diseases is the hantavirus pulmonary syndrome, a severe disease first recognized in 1993 in the USA and now reported from 20 American states and also from Latin America (Schmaljohn & Hjell, 1997: 95; Wells et al. 1997: 171). It is caused by several hantaviruses, one called Sin Nombre, residing principally in deer mice. In several states of the USA after a few years of drought, there was abundant snow and rainfall in the spring of 1993. There was a huge crop of pine kernels, the mice proliferated and, consequently, the risk to humans increased because of contamination of the environment with mice excreta. The disease had probably occurred before but was never recognized as a specific entity. When a doctor saw two 'strange' cases of adult respiratory distress syndrome in young, healthy patients, he became suspicious and searched for other similar, unexplained cases. The laboratory of the Centers for Disease Control and Prevention (CDC), with experience in hantaviruses, was involved, and the cause of this syndrome was quickly found (Garrett 1995).

was traced back to Liberia where a few infected persons were found (WHO 1995b).

In 1995 there was the outbreak in Kikwit, Zaire, very much related to hospital and funeral practices. In total, there were 315 patients with 244 deaths, a case fatality rate of 77% (WHO 1995a). Despite extensive investigations a reservoir was not found, and we do not know how the index case was infected.

In 1996 Ebola appeared in Gabon in people who had butchered and eaten a chimpanzee.[8] There were no hospital-associated secondary cases, and the epidemic was declared over (WHO 1996b). Later in the same year and in the same area, however, Ebola activity reappeared, again related to monkeys. A secondary case, a Gabonese doctor, flew to Johannesburg and survived, but a nurse who cared for him died of Ebola fever (Georges-Courbot et al. 1997; WHO 1996c). In these two outbreaks in Gabon, in total 97 persons fell ill, and 45 died (WHO 1996b, 1997b).

In all these outbreaks the spread of the virus was facilitated by man, perhaps to lesser extent in Gabon. Common factors include: poverty, abysmal medical facilities, poorly paid or unpaid health workers, lack of equipment. Availability of transport was helpful in bringing in needed resources quickly. But it also created a lot of confusion, because people who became scared got as far away as possible from the origin of the outbreak in a short period of time.

Transmission of Ebola virus between men has only been demonstrated via fluids, not via aerosols.[9] This means that control of an epidemic should be rather straightforward and cost little: isolation of patients and care of them with proper measures of wearing cloves, gowns and masks and disposal of excreta, use of disposable materials, and immediate burial of dead bodies without washing and further touching. However, handing over of unwashed dead to the authorities without properly attending to them may be a serious violation of customs and may be met with strong resistance.

Prevention and control of epidemics

Some common causes of the emergence of epidemics

There is a wide range of common causes for the emergence of epidemics including:

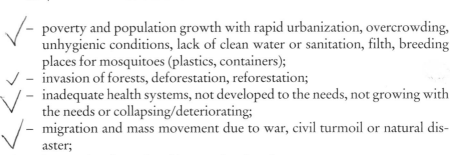

- poverty and population growth with rapid urbanization, overcrowding, unhygienic conditions, lack of clean water or sanitation, filth, breeding places for mosquitoes (plastics, containers);
- invasion of forests, deforestation, reforestation;
- inadequate health systems, not developed to the needs, not growing with the needs or collapsing/deteriorating;
- migration and mass movement due to war, civil turmoil or natural disaster;
- international travel and international trade;
- changes in behaviour (e.g. sexual activities, use of drugs, alcohol, tobacco);
- antimicrobial use and abuse may cause changing patterns of sensitivity of microbial agents to drugs and epidemics due to drug-resistant bacteria.
- Climatic change: due to changes in weather and climate, increases or changes of populations of insects and vectors of disease may occur. Due to change in the sea temperature algae may proliferate, and shellfish poisons may increase. People might move because of climate change, with consequences for the health services. Because of its influence on food crops, climate may be involved in malnutrition and possibly resistance to infections. Ultraviolet light may cause diminished delayed type hypersensitivity response and possibly have other influences on immunity (Patz et al. 1996: 217).

Prevention and control

The *World Health Report 1996* (WHO, 1996a) mentions the following measures in responding to epidemics:
- establishing the diagnosis;
- source investigation;
- control implementation;
- research for means to treat and to prevent spread;
- production of drugs and vaccines;
- establishing a surveillance system;
- promoting an international network of control agencies.

Prevention and control depend on breaking the chain of transmission. To be able to do that, we need to understand this chain. In some instances we still need research into all components of this chain. For example, the reservoir of Ebola virus and Marburg virus and how man becomes infected are unknown. We may still need to develop means to break the chain, for example, vaccines, drugs, insecticides. Public health measures will often be required, like global immunization. Sometimes other interventions are needed (e.g. for dracunculiasis, case detection and sanitation; for the eradication of leprosy, case detection and multidrug treatment). Failure of these measures is not necessarily due to lack of knowledge or tools. It may be due to logistic problems, or to a series of events and developments not infrequently man-made and often poverty-related.

In some of the examples of epidemics given earlier, the causes are evident and measures of prevention and control are easily derived. However, the implementation and sustainability of such measures may be difficult to achieve, for instance, because of the specific combination of causative and contributing factors.

If men would not go into the forest and clear it, they would not come into contact with unknown and possibly dangerous microbial agents (apart

f

h

i

t

f

v

c

r

c

c

a

r

i

r

F

c

c

be
rians
cially rela
lis. The hug
century, peaki
to an explosion o
populations of Chi
Chinese population drop
probably due to plague and
Europe's population, 20 to 30
and 1350, most of them in cities.
citizens, Bremen two-thirds.

Until the early 18th century plague
breaks in Western Europe, mostly in tow
of 24,148 people died, which implies a death ra
1995). The last great plague epidemic in England, t

The historical perspective

Epidemics have been with man since he started his sedentary life, that is, since agrarian society arose (Conrad et al. 1995; McNeill 1976). Have we learned from history? What can we learn from history? In the following outline some important historical developments stand out: urbanization as a major factor in the emergence of large-scale epidemics, and improvement of social and economic conditions as a process leading to their decline.

About 6000 BC the world population of 30 million people lived dispersed over the warmer parts of the globe. By 2000 BC concentration along rivers had occurred and towns of a few thousand people had developed, like Memphis and Thebes. In 60 BC the world population had increased to 300 million. In China and the Roman empire, towns of tens of thousands existed, and by 5 BC Rome was a huge city of 1 million people. London was the first city after Rome to achieve this size, but this only happened in the nineteenth century.

The life expectancy of the population of Rome was far shorter than that in the Mediterranean countryside or in North Africa. In Rome only about 35% of the residents reached the age of 30, while in the countryside 70% did. In town almost no one became 80 years old, while 15% of people living in the countryside did (Garrett 1995: 234-259).

Records from ancient Egypt, Greece, Rome, India, and China tell about the scourges carried by insects in the cities. Chinese records from centuries fore our era report on massive epidemics which arose from cities. Histo-like McNeill (1976) consider four big epidemic plagues as being espe-ted to towns: plague (pneumonic), leprosy, tuberculosis and syphi-e pandemic of plague (the Black Death) in Europe in the 14th between 1346 and 1350, started in Mongolia, possibly due the rodent population due to weather conditions. The India and the Middle East were decimated, the ped from 123 million in 1200 to 65 million in 1393, its aftermath of famine. A quarter to a third of million persons, died of plague between 1346 London and Hamburg lost half of their

continued to cause epidemic out-. In Amsterdam in 1664, a total te of 120 per thousand (Israel e Great Plague of London

(1665), was probably stopped by the Great Fire of 1666 that destroyed a large part of the town with its wooden houses and thatch roofs, nice refuges for rats. Brick houses and tiles replaced the old constructions, producing fewer contacts between men, fleas and rodents. In most of Western Europe, stone and brick houses with tile roofs became the standard, not so much because of hygienic considerations but because of a shortage of wood. Another important factor in the disappearance of plague was the gradual replacement of the black rat by the brown rat (the sewer rat) with other habits of living, and less close to man.

Why plague disappeared from Western Europe long before the advent of antibiotics and long before its exact cause and transmission were known is not completely resolved. We also do not know why leprosy died out in Western Europe with the advent of the Black Death. Leprosy may not be a very old disease, as no signs of it are found in skeletons prior to 500 AD (Garrett 1995). Leprosy entered the Mediterranean area and Europe in the sixth century and spread and increased in number in parallel with the rise of cities up to the 14th century. Tuberculosis replaced leprosy as a disease in Western Europe after the Black Death; whether this was causal to the disappearance of leprosy remains unsolved. Evidence of tuberculosis goes back to 5000 BC (Garrett 1995).

Conditions in European cities of the fifteenth to nineteenth century, notably the overcrowding, were favourable for the transmission of the tubercle bacillus. The same was true for towns in North America and South African townships. In 1830 the crude death rate in Boston was 21 per thousand, half that of London; by 1850 it had increased to 38 per thousand. Tuberculosis was a major contributor. From 1830 cholera added to the urban death toll, four pandemics raged around the world between 1830 and 1896. At the peak of the Industrial Revolution, birth rates in the cities were lower than the death rates.

From about 1850 changes gradually occurred in society: improvement of hygiene, cleaning of towns and garbage collection, clean water supply, toilets, reduction of child labour, reduction of working hours, public schools, a public health system, hospitals. In Europe and the USA these developments led to an increase in birth rates, reduction in death rate and increase in life expectancy from about 1900. The incidence of infectious diseases and of death due to these diseases, including tuberculosis, declined, and this long before vaccines and antibiotics were available. For example, in towns in the USA, mortality due to tuberculosis was 200 per 100,000 per year in 1900. It was reduced to 60 per 100,000 by 1940.

It would be useful for developing countries to know how this happened and what was most important in this development. What was the contribution of improvement in nutrition or in housing, of education? Were changes at the workplace and in the working conditions important or changes in the circumstances of daily life? What was the contribution of doctors and the health care system?

Demographic, social and economic developments were probably the most important aspects and led to a reduction of the influence of the big plagues long before modern biotechnological medicine could contribute. If the medical sector played a role, it was in the field of public health (McNeill 1976; Sagan 1987; Conrad et al. 1995).

The contributions of medicine, of the health sector and of individual doctors should, however, not be completely discarded and forgotten. The work of Snow on cholera is an example in case. The control of smallpox in the second half of the nineteenth century was mainly due to vaccination, a technological achievement, and to isolation of patients, and no longer mainly due to social developments. Thorough knowledge of the epidemiology, regularly updated by field studies, played a crucial role in the final eradication of this disease (Coutinho 1989).

In conclusion

Regarding epidemics we are facing relatively new problems, and also old problems in a new context. Important elements of this context are:
- drug-resistant bacteria and parasites, due to increasing use of drugs, to use of subtherapeutic doses, to counterfeit drugs;
- changes in lifestyles and behaviour (e.g. use of narcotics);
- changes in social values and sexual practices;
- increasing international travel and trade.
- adverse effects of modern medical practice: e.g. an increase in the number of cases of viral hepatitis; more immunosuppression and immunodeficiency and consequences thereof;
- new animal diseases like BSE, diseases that have consequences for man. BSE is probably not the last one.

The story of the hantavirus pulmonary syndrome is an example of the type of attitude, the knowledge, the resources, and the infrastructure we need to face new and well-known epidemic challenges. The doctor who saw two young people in perfectly good health die from adult respiratory distress of unknown cause thought that this was odd. He started further investigations, the specialized laboratory of CDC was involved, which has extensive high-tech experience regarding many exotic diseases and their causative agents. Within a few days the cause of death of these young patients, a new virus, was detected. Extensive further investigations uncovered the source.

First, the problem was recognized, and a solution was sought (critical attitude, open and inquisitive mind, perseverance). Then knowledge and expertise brought solutions (education, training, means, infrastructure).

To understand and address the future problems of epidemics, the contribution of people with different academic backgrounds is needed: social, psychological, anthropological, historical, biological and health sciences, inluding veterinarians. They need continuous education and a critical attitude. Many need to be involved in research.

Given the pivotal role which medical institutions play in the treatment, but sometimes also the spreading of epidemics, appropriate guidelines for clinics and hospitals are mandatory, with instructions on how to use and apply them, supervision, regular evaluation and updating. In addition, hospitals and clinics need proper supplies.

For an individual, contributions may seem futile in view of the size of the problems. Yet contributions start from individuals. Individuals make their political choices and have their influence in their social circles. Health workers should not smoke cigarettes and should stimulate people to stop smoking. This will help mitigate the effects of the smoking epidemic. We should try to contribute in our professional life, in giving an example, in teaching and training wherever and whenever we can, in being critical and by stimulating people to be critical, by creating and stimulating a critical and research-minded atmosphere, involving young people of all scientific fields.

Epidemics will always be with us, new and old ones, with new and old agents. Knowledge and experience can prevent panic and will help us with control and prevention. Medicine and the health care sector will play their modest but indisputable role in this concerted action.

Notes

1 It would be appropriate to discuss smoking, probably the most rapidly spreading epidemic, the one epidemic that is actively and aggressively promoted, a man-made epidemic. Cigarette smoking causes 3 million deaths annually, at

present 2/3 of them in the developed world. By the year 2020 cigarette smoking may kill more people than any single disease and if present trends continue smoking is expected to kill 10 million people per year by 2025, 7 million of those in developing countries (Jenkins et al. 1997: 1726).

2   We see this picture, with nuances, also at the local level. McLarty et al. (1996: 247) reported that in Hai District, Northern Tanzania, in adults 60% of the deaths were due to non communicable diseases when HIV infection was excluded. Of these 20% were injuries. When HIV infection was included, non-communicable diseases still accounted for 40% of the death toll.

3   Important sources of infections, also of new infections and epidemics, are our food and water. *Cryptosporidium* appeared as an important cause of diarrhoea. For example in 1993 in Milwaukee, Wisconsin, a break in the public water supply caused an enormous epidemic with more than 400 000 sick people and 4 000 hospitalizations (WHO 1996a).

Cholera was not new to South America; it was absent for almost a century. It is now back and will probably remain for many years to come. The new strain of cholera in South East Asia, *Vibrio cholerae* O139 has the potential of causing a new pandemic (WHO 1996a).

Escherichia coli OH157, contaminating meat, especially hamburgers, caused large outbreaks of bloody diarrhoea in Japan and Scotland (WHO 1997a).

4   Malaria has also been called a 'submerged' disease (Olliaro et al. 1996: 230).

5   In Mauritania a comparable situation occurred in 1987, with a smaller epidemic.

6   S. Halstead in his Special Lecture at the 14th International Conference on Tropical Medicine and Malaria, Nagasaki 1996.

7   In Italy also monkeys from the Philippines died of an Ebola virus.

8   In 1994 some cases had already occurred in Gabon (Georges-Courbot et al. 1997).

9   Airborne transmission has been observed in the monkey facility in the USA, but not so far in man.

Literature

Anonymous
   1996   'Editorial policy and call for articles.' *Emerging infectious diseases* 2(3).
Benenson, A.S.
   1990   *Control of communicable diseases in man.* Washington: American Public Health Association. [Fifteenth ed.]
Centers for Disease Control
   1988   'Management of patients with suspected viral hemorrhagic fever.' *Morbidity and mortality weekly report* 37(S-3): 1-16.

Clegg, J.C.S.
1984 'Possible approaches to a vaccine against Lassa fever.' *Transactions of the Royal Society of Tropical Medicine and Hygiene* 78(2): 307-310.

Conrad, L.I., M. Neve, V. Nutton, R. Porte & A. Wear
1995 *The western medical tradition. 800 BC to AD 1800.* Cambridge: Cambridge University Press.

Coutinho, R.A.
1989 *Van pokken, syphilis en AIDS. Geschiedenis van de infectieziektenbestrijding door de eeuwen heen.* Amsterdam: De Bij.

Ekwanzala, M., J. Pepin, N. Khonde, S. Molisho, H. Bruneel & P. De Wals
1996 'In the heart of darkness: sleeping sickness in Zaire.' *Lancet* 348(22): 1427-1430.

Fisher-Hoch, S.P., O. Tomori, A. Nasidi, G.I. Perez-Oronoz, Y. Fakile, L. Hutwagner & J.B.M. McCormick
1995 'Review of cases of nosocomial Lassa fever in Nigeria: the price of poor medical practice.' *British Medical Journal* 311(14): 857-859.

Garrett, L.
1995 *The coming plague.* London: Virago Press.

Georges-Courbet, M.C., A. Sanchez, C.Y. Lu, S. Baize, E. Leroy, J. Lansout-Soukate, C. Tévi-Benissan, A.J. Georges, S.G. Trappier, S.R. Zaki, R. Swanepoel, P.A. Leman, P.E. Rollin, C.J. Peters, S.T. Nichol & T.G. Ksiazek
1997 'Isolation and phylogenetic characterization of Ebola viruses causing different outbreaks in Gabon.' *Emerging Infectious Diseases* 3(1): 59-62.

Helmick, C.G., P.A. Webb, C.L. Scribner, J.W. Krebs & J.B. McCormick
1986 'No evidence for increased risk of lassa fever infection in hospital staff.' *Lancet* 328 (21): 1202-1205.

Israel, J.I.
1995 *The Dutch Republic. Its rise, greatness and fall 1477-1806.* Oxford: Clarendon Press.

Jenkins, C.N.H., P.X. Dai, D.H. Ngoc, H.V. Kinh, T.T. Hoang, S. Bales, S. Stewart & S.J. McPhee
1997 'Tobacco use in Vietnam. Prevalence, predictors, and the role of the transnational tobacco corporations.' *JAMA* 277(21): 1726-1731.

Le Guenno, B., P. Formentry, M. Wyers, P. Gounon, F. Walker & C. Boesch
1995 'Isolation and partial characterisation of a new strain of Ebola virus.' *Lancet* 345 (20): 1271-1274.

Le Guenno, B.
1995 'Emerging viruses.' *Scientific American*, October 1995, pp. 30-37.

Louria, D.B.
1996 'Emerging and re-emerging infections: the societal variables.' *International Journal of Infectious Disease* 1(2): 59-62.

McNeill, W.H.
    1976   *Plagues and peoples*. Harmondsworth: Penguin Books.
McLarty, D., K.G.M.M., Alberti & N. Unwin
    1996   'Tropical medicine should become specialty of "health in developing countries".' *British Medical Journal* 312(4): 247-248.
Olliaro, P., J. Cattani & D. Wirth
    1996   'Malaria, the submerged disease.' *JAMA* 275(3): 230-233.
Patz, J.A., P.R. Epstein, T.A. Burke & J.M. Balbus
    1996   'Global climate change and emerging infectious diseases.' *JAMA* 275(3): 217-223.
Peters, C.J., A. Sanchez, H. Feldmann, P.E. Rollin, S. Nichol & T.G. Ksiazek
    1994   'Filovirus as emerging pathogens.' *Seminars in Virology* 5(1): 147-154.
Sagan, L.A.
    1987   *The health of nations. True causes of sickness and well-being*. New York: Basic Books.
Schmaljohn, C. & B. Hjell
    1997   'Hantaviruses: A global disease problem.' *Emerging Infectious Diseases* 3(2): 95-103.
Wells, R.M., S.S. Estani, Z.E. Yadon, D. Enria, P. Padula, N. Pini, J.N. Mills, C.J. Peters & E.L. Segura
    1997   'An unusual Hantavirus outbreak in Southern Argentina: Person to person transmission?' *Emerging Infectious Diseases* 3(2): 171-174.
World Health Organization
    1995a   'Ebola haemorrhagic fever.' *Weekly Epidemiological Record* 70(34): 241-242.
    1995b   'Ebola haemorrhagic fever. Confirmed case in Cote d'Ivoire and suspect case in Liberia.' *Weekly Epidemiological Record* 70(50): 359.
    1996a   *The World Health Report 1996*. Geneva: WHO.
    1996b   'Outbreak of Ebola haemorrhagic fever in Gabon officially declared over.' *Weekly Epidemiological Record* 71(17): 125-126.
    1996c   'Ebola haemorrhagic fever.' *Weekly Epidemiological Record* 71(47): 359.
    1997a   *The World Health Report 1997*. Geneva: WHO.
    1997b   'Ebola haemorrhagic fever.' *Weekly Epidemiological Record* 72(10): 71.

CHAPTER 2

Project for a Beneficial Epidemic: On the Collective Aspects of Contagion and Prevention[1]

ABRAM DE SWAAN

Sometimes it takes a disaster to prod people into action which they had refrained from taking until then out of ignorance, indifference or lack of confidence in their peers. Thus, preventive measures are usually adopted only when the catastrophe they are supposed to prevent has already occurred, once. Usually, the discussion centres about the question of what should be done to make sure that disaster will not strike again. Here, I will ask the reverse question: What kind of catastrophe does it take before people will adopt the policies that would have been feasible and beneficial all along? More precisely, the question is, what kind of medical emergency would persuade the authorities in the wealthy countries of the world to act collectively in order to improve public health conditions in the poor countries of the globe?

Posing the question by no means implies wishing for the event. The purpose is a thought experiment that may demonstrate the connections between the dynamics of major epidemics, on the one hand, and the adoption of large-scale public health and social policies on the other.

The starting point is past experience, especially the history of the nineteenth century cholera epidemics and the subsequent implementation of the municipal sanitary measures that turned out to be most effective. At a later stage, national governments put in place health policies on a countrywide scale. At present, environmental and health risks operate on a global scale and are a matter of worldwide concern. However, so far it has proved very difficult to coordinate preventive and remedial policies on the corresponding world scale. The theory of the collectivizing process (De Swaan 1988), which explains the emergence (and the absence) of collective arrangements to remedy adversities and deficiencies on an adequate scale, will guide the argument.

Cholera in nineteenth century Europe

When early in the nineteenth century cholera appeared in Western Europe, it was widely interpreted in the Biblical tradition as a Divine Plague sent in punishment for the multifarious sins of city-dwellers (Finer 1952). By the middle of the nineteenth century, enlightened public opinion had come to see it somewhat differently: cholera was considered God's judgement on the poor for neglecting His sanitary laws. Medical men and administrators increasingly came to believe that cholera spread because of ill vapors, miasma, exuding from stagnant polluted pools and humid, dark dwellings where neither sunlight or fresh air ever penetrated. This 'miasmatic' view stood in stark opposition to the 'contagionist' opinion that sick persons carried some invisible agent that caused the disease and which they could pass on to others (Pelling 1961). Its opponents considered the contagionist view outdated, reactionary, and even worse, Roman Catholic, since it had inspired such fiendish measures as the *quarantine* which was still practised in the backward port cities of the Mediterranean (La Berge 1974). Indeed, for centuries plagues had triggered drastic intervention by the authorities: isolation of suspected patients, burning of their household possessions, destruction of incoming merchandise and a ban on exporting goods, a strict prohibition on entering or leaving the town, etc. Carlo Cipolla's beautiful account (1979) of bubonic plague epidemics during the seventeenth century shows vividly how extreme and often how counterproductive these desperate remedies could be: massive prayer meetings in the afflicted towns certainly caused the sick to infect the healthy.

The hygienists would have nothing to do with the antiquated superstitions they ascribed to the contagionists; they were men of science, doctors, engineers, administrators, and they knew how to eradicate miasma, wherever they suspected it (Murard & Zylberman 1985). They proposed to combat the bad vapors by a massive cleaning campaign in the poorer parts of town. Stagnant pools and canals had to be drained, unsanitary dwellings were to be evacuated, if necessary with police coercion, and the slums with their dark alleys and filthy courts were to be pulled down. Stray animals, dogs, goats, pigs and chickens that roamed the streets had to be rounded up. All garbage was to be collected several times a week. And that was not all: '*Tout á l'égout*', everything into the sewers, became the rallying cry of the Parisian hygienist reformers (Goubert 1986; Kalff 1995). Theirs was an ambitious scheme indeed. In order to deal once and for all with the looming threat of cholera, the entire city should be rinsed daily with clean water to take away the filth and absorb the rains so as to prevent pools from forming, and this cleansing stream should also carry with it all household sewerage and human excrements.

In line with this grand scheme, the great Parisian sewer system was constructed, one of the most outstanding engineering feats of the century. In London, Sir Edwin Chadwick went even further in designing what he called the great 'venal-arterial system', taking his cue from the model of blood circulation (Finer 1952): fresh drinking water was to be pumped into the city and distributed through a network of ever finer branches into every household; there it was to be used for drinking, cooking and washing. In each home, the waste water of kitchen, bath and toilet would be collected and transported through small sewer pipes by way of increasingly larger branches into canals leading out of the city, into the river and into the sea.

This same vision of the city as an immense organism was further elaborated by Von Liebig, who proposed collecting human waste from every dwelling, carrying it to a processing plant and turning it into manure, which could then be used to fertilize the soil of the surrounding farmlands, which in turn would produce the crops to feed the urban citizens. Another perfect cycle, this time of nutrition, digestion, secretion and fertilization.

In 1856, during a cholera outbreak in London, the physician John Snow discovered a hearth of infection, the notorious Broadstreet pump: it turned out that all cholera patients in the area had drunk its water before they came down with the disease. This was strong evidence for the contagionist view; but the discovery of the actual disease agent *Vibrio cholera* by Pacini in 1854 was largely ignored until Koch rediscovered it in 1883 and finally decided the controversy in favor of the contagionists. In the meantime the hygienists had succeeded in pushing through their sanitary reforms, not only Chadwick in London or Villermé and Parent-Duchatelet in Paris, but also Virchow in Berlin, Liernur in Amsterdam, Shattuck in Boston and Von Pettenkofer in Munich.

Of course, the world famous Professor Pettenkofer had refuted the alleged causal connection between contaminated water and cholera *ex cathedra*, in front of a learned audience, by emptying in one gulp a glass of water said to contain the lethal contaminant. He survived his feat in good health, most likely because he was so excited and angry during his performance that his stomach held enough acid to kill the cholera bacteria on the spot.

The hygienists, the doctors, the engineers and the great administrators were staunchly convinced that 'the only real contribution of medicine to civilization was the sanitary and hygienic regulations it had helped to institute.' Rosenberg (1962) adds that they believed these measures to be worth more than all 'the drugs of Galen and Paracelsus combined. It was 1865 and the miracle drugs of Roche and Pfizer were yet undiscovered.'

Tirelessly the reformers campaigned for their great sanitary schemes, and with hindsight it can be said that they did the right thing for the wrong reasons. Clean drinking water, sound sewers and, it should be added, uncontaminated milk and meat (Koolmees 1997) did not only help to put an end to the urban scourge of cholera, they may well have been the most important scientific contribution ever to the general health of the population (McKeown 1976).

Rarely has the irony of history, what Hegel has called 'the ruse of reason', been so tellingly revealed as in the episode that pitched the contagionists and the adherents of the miasma theory against each other. The latter stuck to their convictions about the evil vapors of the city and continued to dominate the discussion. And yet, for the wrong reasons, they kept on pushing the right policies: the great cleansing of urban squalor that did so much damage to the citizens' health.

The misunderstandings among the hygienists of the day were in fact most productive. The heroic era of the hygienists brought about the radical collectivization of disease prevention through the creation of an effective public health system.

Somewhat ruefully, Barbara Rosenkrantz (1972: 192) concludes that by the end of the nineteenth century the focus of medicine began to shift from collective sanitary measures toward the treatment of individual patients, as new diagnostic methods and curative techniques became available, dealing with one patient at a time. Medicine increasingly abandoned collective concerns and occupied itself with the individual patient. By that time, in most Western cities urban sanitary installations and public health services had been put in place.

Urban squalor was the concomitant of poverty. It was the curse of 'the great unwashed', as the British called 'the other half': the poor. It was commonly held that badly ventilated, dark and damp spaces, such as the poor dwelled in, exuded these evil vapors. The stagnant water in gutters and pools, the garbage lying about everywhere, the excrements in dark corners and obscure stairwells and courts, all the filth of the slums, were considered a threat to the health of the poor and, indirectly, of everyone else in the city. The specter of cholera transformed this concern for the poor into something much larger, into a pervasive anxiety among all citizens for their own health and well-being. The menace transformed the afflictions of individual poor people into a generalized threat for everyone.

In other words, in economic terms, it externalized the effects of one person's adversity and deficiency into a collective danger for everyone in the city and its surroundings. That is the perverse blessing of contagion. The perception of these external effects, which did not even spare the rich, was what motivated the profound and incisive urban sanitary reforms: clean and running drinking water under constant pressure, a steady stream of sewage carried away by a system of pipes, the continuous cleaning of the streets, the regular collection of garbage, and finally the construction of public schools and workers' houses where daylight and fresh air could freely enter.

With hindsight, this enormous programme of sanitary reform was not really necessary to effectively combat cholera or other contagious diseases. Even at the time, protection on an individual basis or in single households would have been possible. If common toilets had been kept clean, if hands were washed before each meal, fresh vegetables and fruit rinsed before eating, bottled water consumed (or if people would have restricted themselves to beer which was consumed also for its purity), and if people would have stayed away from their poorest and filthiest fellow citizens and forced their domestic servants to abide by the same regime, they might have avoided infection. Moreover, the general health of the privileged classes was such that they did not easily succumb to infectious disease such as cholera, and even if they came down with it, they usually survived the attack, children and the elderly excepted. But it was precisely the specter of cholera, the mystified and magnified nightmare of intractable evil vapors, of mortal miasma, this vague, diffuse and omnipresent danger that threatened each and everyone, that helped convince the established burghers of the city, the respectable bourgeoisie, who after all had to pay the taxes and finance the sanitary measures, to support the grand scheme of the great reformers: the image of the city as one circulatory organism, as a single digestive process. The organicist vision of the urban population as one huge, interdependent whole helped to transform the urban body politic in fact into a more coherent entity, ready to undertake the collective measures that might subdue the common danger.

These reforms were realized in England, Germany, France, the USA, the Netherlands and elsewhere during the heyday of liberalism, when the doctrine of government abstentionism, of the nightwatch state, was at its zenith. Nevertheless, a 'municipal socialism' or 'a gas and water socialism' prevailed in many cities of Europe. It should be added that the innovations served the urban developers quite well: in the new residential areas, the presence of water closets, sewers, and a constant supply of running water were an excellent sales argument to the new bourgeois who bought these houses. For the first time, people could live in surroundings that did not smell of faeces. And soon, the evil fragrance of human waste became a tell-tale sign of poverty and a social embarrassment to boot. In the process, a possibility that was initially limited to the happy few, soon became a necessity for everyone: not to be confronted and put to shame by the sight and smell of excrement (Gleichman 1979; Vigarello 1985).

In the course of some 50 years, defecation and excrement that had always been a token of human presence became imperceptible to others. As a result, everything having to do with human waste disappeared from conversation and, in good part, from consciousness. Scatological jokes and worries have become much less common than they were a century ago. As the intricate web of pipes and drains spread underground, the concern with human filth and waste was relegated to the subconscious. It continued as a preoccupation only for young children who were yet to be toilet trained, and for some adults it became the 'anal' obsession soon to be rediscovered by Sigmund Freud in the fantasies of ailing neurotics. In the sprawling shantytowns of Asia and Africa, where as yet no adequate sanitary provisions have been installed, the scenes and odours of defecation still are familiar (although passersby will ostentatiously ignore them) and the smell of open sewers often pervades the poor areas, very much as it did in the nineteenth century cities of the West.

The dynamics of urban sanitary reforms

Much has been left out of this account, admittedly a greatly simplified and highly idealized version of the great nineteenth century urban revolution in public hygiene. Malaria was not mentioned, nor tuberculosis and venereal diseases, over the years much greater killers than cholera during its brief appearances. I have not discussed the formidable opposition of landlords who resented the inspection by the medical police and refused to carry the costs of sanitary improvement. I mention only in passing our forebears' peculiar obsessions with their excrement, which they did not want to abandon to the dark sewers, since after all it represented useful manure, nor did they trust the anonymous municipal authorities with their intimate excrement which, who knows, might be used against them. I will not elaborate on the rage of the poor who were wont to believe that cholera was the result of a conspiracy by the rich to kill them off so as to relieve the burden of the poor tax, or their resistance against the demolition of their wretched homes and familiar slums, the elimination of the goats and pigs they relied on for food, or the closing down of the small workshops where they made their meager living.

What matters here primarily is how did this great municipal reform come about? What were its social and political dynamics? It was a prime example of a collectivizing process: a historical episode in which the enlightened citizens came to realize that the adversities and deficiencies that afflict the poor in their midst carry external effects that also threaten them, the rich. Once they became aware of this interdependence between their lives and those of the poor, they were more willing to take measures so as to ward off these threats. The main problem to be solved next was to ensure the compliance of their peers and distribute the costs among them. That – in a nutshell – is the theory of the collectivizing process that gave the impetus to the creation of care arrangements on an ever increasing scale, from poor relief in the medieval parish to public sanitation in the nineteenth century city, and to the twentieth century welfare state of nationwide scope (de Swaan 1988).

The evil vapors that exuded from the slums did threaten the rich collectively. Wealthy citizens could not put an end to this danger by their own individual efforts, they had to coordinate their actions. Yet, some of their number might be unwilling to contribute to the common effort and nevertheless profit without any sacrifice on their part. This mutual suspicion is familiar in all episodes where collective action is required. It evokes the notorious dilemma: I can profit without collaborating; but if many others likewise refuse to cooperate, nothing will happen, and all of us will be worse off. On the other hand, if I join with others in the collective effort and it succeeds, some may profit from it without cost. There are several ways out of this dilemma. Here only one is germane: external coercion. That provided in fact the dynamics of urban sanitary reform. There was already a strong and effective metropolitan government that could enforce its policies upon hesitant citizens, impose its taxes on willing or reluctant contributors, demand access for its inspectors and exact compliance to the orders of its medical police. And so it happened.

In this particular case, a system of sewers and water supply, the provisions that were installed, did not constitute a purely collective or public good: the systems consisted of networks of pipes and tubes, all coming together in a central installation with pumps and purification plants for drinking water or sewerage treatment (Van Zon 1986; Van den Noort 1990). Private companies were granted a license to build the central plants and the networks for fresh water supply and the collection of waste water. They could then connect private subscribers individually and collect a fee from them. The new, wealthy residential districts were the first to be connected. Once the central installations had been put in place and the main pipes in the course of time crossed the greater part of the city, it became easier and cheaper to provide services in the older areas and to supply the poor at low cost or with a municipal grant (the study of Tilburg by Van der Heijden 1994, 1995a, b corroborates these findings, but the author remains quite skeptical). This circumstance, the 'network structure' of the arrangement, greatly facilitated its acceptance by the taxpayers and its gradual extension throughout the nineteenth century city.

Even though the systems, once in place, could be operated on a commercial footing, their very scale and monopolistic character required support and regulation from the municipal authorities. The provisions came about because the better-off citizens believed they too were endangered by the ills that afflicted the poor in their cities. In order words, the rich were aware of the interdependence between themselves and the destitute city-dwellers. That was the lesson they learned from the urban plague, from cholera, and although their reasons were misguided, their remedies turned out to be most efficacious.

Global interdependencies

This argument has analogies that apply directly to the contemporary predicament, and with a vengeance. The interdependence between the various parts of the globe has increased spectacularly. The nineteenth century question of urban sanitation was of course an ecological matter, a problem of environmental pollution that went by a different – medical – name and operated on another, more restricted scale. Nowadays, the informed public is well aware of the global implications of environmental disturbances: how air pollution in China affects the pine woods in Norway, how a nuclear accident in Chernobyl contaminates the harvest in Italy, how the destruction of the rain forests of Indonesia may change the climate in the usa.

The concept of externalities, of collective goods, or rather collective evils, is uncannily familiar, and once again the dilemmas of collective action exercise their paralysing influence. Why should one country limit its discharge of carbon dioxyde, if other countries continue to pollute the air with the fumes from their traffic and factories? City governments could coordinate action on the urban scale, but presently there is no world government that can effectively coordinate the 190 states in the world, in order to limit environmental pollution and punish those states that remain uncooperative and might profit from a cleaner environment without restricting their own discharges. However, people are much less accustomed to consider public health problems on this global scale as a subject for worldwide collective action. So far, medical prevention is mostly a matter of health services operating as government agencies on a national level.

Yet, the scale of infectious epidemics has been transcontinental and even global for many centuries already: contagion spread with the trading caravans across deserts and seas. It came with invading armies from the Far East to the West where millions succumbed to germs against which they had not yet acquired resistance. Next, European conquerors brought diseases to the Americas where the indigenous population had not developed immunity against them (cf. McNeill 1976; see also contributions Kager and Streefland, this volume). The global scale of epidemics is not unprecedented, but their travelling speed has now increased by a factor of one hundred, or more. Contemporary germs move by jet instead of camel and donkey, their carriers travel not by dozens but by the thousands, even millions. An infectious disease that erupts anywhere on this earth represents a danger of contagion for people everywhere else on the globe. If people are at all aware of this global and immediate interdependency, of the reach and speed of these external effects of disease, they often react defensively and opt for measures of exclusion. In their fear, and often further excited by the mass media, they may even exaggerate the dangers. So far, these anxieties have not prompted support for positive measures of prevention at the danger sites themselves, along the lines of the nineteenth century urban sanitation campaigns.

Contemporary conditions of production and distribution have on the one hand improved the bacterial and chemical purity of food and medication, but the very same circumstances have also created new risks, with a vast potential impact. One hundred years ago, the great majority of people on this earth lived on the land and consumed the food they themselves had produced. One cow fed one family, with a few relatives and neighbors. Today, in the developed world only a tiny minority grows and eats its own food, and even in the developing world the self-feeding rural population is rapidly dwindling. Cattle and poultry are raised by the thousands, slaughtered by the millions, and their meat is processed in large plants and distributed to tens of millions of consumers. As a consequence, a single hearth of infection may affect many millions of consumers. Nor is it only food that is distributed so widely, but also medication and blood products. The plasma of thousands of donors was centrally collected and processed, the product distributed to many thousands of patients, and administered to some of them not once, but ten, twenty times a year, year after year. Even as this went on, it was known that there might be contaminants that went unnoticed at the time as they could not be identified by the available methods. With hindsight it can be said that this meant courting disaster. And disaster duly arrived: the infection of haemophiliacs with hiv through mass-produced blood-based medication. It may be argued that the risk was worth the gain, a sustainable life for the sufferers of haemophilia. As it happens, it is particularly difficult to make risk assessments of very small odds for a very large number of events. But the pros and cons were probably never rationally assessed; the dangers were simply ignored.

With bovine spongiform encephalopathy something similar occurred in Western Europe. Probably, for the first time in the many millions of years of the history of the bovine species, cattle was fed with animal remains. No one knew, no one could know, no one knows even now what risks were involved in the introduction of this new fodder. But again, if a single animal develops some condition that is contagious and harmful to human beings, this one source of contaminated meat may reach untold numbers of consumers through the vast networks of industrial processing and commercial distribution. In this case, also, no one knew the risks involved, and no risk assessment of this new feeding method seems to have been tried: a clear case of veterinary arrogance, commercial greed and official negligence. Even when measures were finally taken, they were evaded on a large scale with the connivance of the authorities. At present, the scare seems to have blown over without too many casualties, but given the wide distribution of contaminated meat over a number of years and the very long incubation period of the disease, the outcome is by no means certain, and a public health disaster may still be in the offing. The most recent veterinary outburst, a persistent epidemic of swine fever, this time in the Netherlands, proceeded again along the same lines, when semen used in mass artificial insemination turned out, against all expert opinion, to transfer the virus.

The recent episodes of contaminated food and medication represent an old drama blown up to the scale of contemporary production, distribution and consumption on a mass scale. These events are not incidental epiphenomena but, on the contrary, are a direct consequence of the highly centralized manufacture and very widely dispersed use of the products involved. There is a clear pattern in these instances of mass contamination that is likely to occur again and again along similar lines. Since markets now span the continents and encompass the entire globe, inspection and regulation must reach as far. However, even the European Union, at present the most effective supranational agency, has proved incapable of exerting adequate control. On the other hand, consumer reaction has been very strong and resulted in buyers' strikes that caused considerable loss to suppliers. Here, again, a dilemma of collective action operates, since the sector as a whole stands to lose from these incidents, whereas individual firms may profit by evading regulations. In this case, too, the solution must come from diligent inspection and active enforcement of strict rules by an authority that functions on an adequate scale, i.e. with a continental or even global reach.

Epidemic interdependencies between rich and poor countries

The main line of the present argument concerns the external effects of contagion in a somewhat different context, one which implies an interdependence between the rich and the poor. In the modern world, where such externalities operate swiftly over very large distances, this primarily refers to the interdependence between the inhabitants of the richer countries and those of the poorer areas of the world. What sorts of diseases that afflict the indigent inhabitants of faraway lands might affect the citizens of the wealthier areas? And if such diseases do indeed occur there, to what extent is Western public opinion aware of the externalities they bring about? Finally, one might ask, under what conditions is it conceivable that awareness of these external effects will prompt collective action on behalf of the richer nations so as to minimize the threats of epidemic disease that they involve? Is it conceivable that anything like the great sanitary reforms of the nineteenth century cities could be initiated in order to control the threats of contagion that disease among the poor of this world may cause for its richer inhabitants?

Apart from the risks of contaminated food and medicine, which still derive mainly from the rich world itself, there are at least two major epidemiological hazards which quite often have their origin in the poorer parts of the globe. The first is the emergence of new varieties of infectious and harmful micro-organisms that are resistant to drugs, not just one kind of drug, but sometimes all known remedies. Malaria and tuberculosis, but also gonorrhoea, are cases in point; other instances of drug-resistant germs, for example, streptococcus, are encountered in today's hospitals. Many of these resistant varieties emerged in countries where antibiotics and other drugs are routinely given without proper diagnostic testing, where there is no medical personnel to supervise treatment so as to make sure that patients complete their course, or where contraband drugs, often far beyond their expiration date, are freely available over the counter or in open air markets, without any medical prescription or supervision. Medication administered in this manner serves not to immunize the patient but to breed immune strains of the contaminant (Van der Geest, this volume; Kager, this volume). The same happens in Western countries, where in the inner cities many people, uprooted or deranged, do not care to finish their courses of treatment as prescribed and cannot be made to do so (unless properly supervised). Moreover, all sorts of antibiotics, pesticides, hormones and other drugs are added to meat and produce, equally contributing to the emergence of drug-resistant varieties of microparasites.

Having survived their encounter with greatly weakened medicine, at lower doses and for shorter periods, these new strains are further selected until they are fully resistant against the most advanced treatment methods and can withstand every available remedy. Moreover, these new specimens travel fast and far, wherever their carriers will bring them with trains, cars and airplanes. In advanced societies, government regulations are adopted that limit the abuse of medical drugs and prevent the emergence of resistant strains. States can impose effective controls within the confines of their territory, and they can even coordinate their efforts to a degree by treaty and through international organizations. But government controls in non-Western countries are much less efficacious, and authorities there hesitate to limit the choices of citizens who have just begun to taste the fruits of modern medicine. However, contagion or contamination that originates in those countries does not stop at the borders of Western states. Once again, the problem has many features of a collective action predicament, this time at the global level.

The second epidemiological threat that partly originates in the poor countries of this world is that of newly emerging diseases, either entirely new to the human species or reactivated after long periods of latency (McCaa 1996). In many instances, the spread of these new microbial species is due to iatrogenic causes: injection by septic needles, infection from one patient to another (Garrett 1994). Bloodborne infections do not spread all that easily through a population as long as nurses, doctors and dentists do not help them along, and this form of contagion does not easily cross state borders. Sexual transmission may be another route, as in the case of hepatitis, HIV and the classical sexually transmitted diseases. In this case, individuals may rely on their own resources to protect themselves:

by using condoms, abstaining from sex or by being cautious in selecting partners and practices.

People can also protect themselves against diseases that spread by contaminated or spoiled food, if they are warned duly and in time. The same goes for waterborne infections. Thus, what characteristics should a disease have to bring about the kind of situation that cholera created in nineteenth-century cities, but this time on a world scale, and against all expertise and resources presently available?

The contagious agent should be airborne, since such infection is the hardest for individuals to protect themselves against. It should not cause any detectable symptoms in the first days or weeks, while being fully infectious from the outset. This would make it very hard to isolate carriers or to protect oneself from them. Moreover, no individual means of prevention or treatment should be available. And, of course, the disease should be very harmful, if not lethal (killing its own host in the process). In many respects, it should be like influenza. In fact, the Spanish flu of 1918-1919 (McNeill 1976: 288-9) was one of the worst epidemics ever to afflict humanity. But the Spanish flu came and went too quickly to prompt collective initiatives on the required, global scale. The ideal epidemic therefore should continue for some years so as to allow governments and international organizations the time to overcome their dilemmas and effectively coordinate their actions.

Obviously, aids was a very good try at a worldwide epidemic that might have prompted a global sanitary campaign, but it spread in ways not useful to terrorize the general public. [It did however prompt homosexuals to organize themselves, protest stigmatization and create not only – collective – action groups demanding funding for research and treatment, but also to establish a host of arrangements for mutual care through collective action.]

But neither in the case of Spanish flu nor in hiv did the public perceive a clear causal connection with poverty. So, the imaginary epidemic should be broadly perceived as originating under conditions of poverty, and as very likely to spread – by air quickly and inexorably over very large distances, never sparing the rich on its fateful course. A new, virulent strain of tuberculosis would make the most suitable candidate for an epidemic that might elicit preventive action on a global scale.

Such a plague would persuade the governments and the international organizations that massive intervention was required in order to improve the conditions of the poor wherever the disease was endemic. If states could succeed in overcoming their dilemmas of collective action, they would embark on a collective campaign to fight poverty in those faraway countries.

In current discussions the problem of global poverty is discussed more and more in connection with worldwide environmental problems, under the heading of 'sustainable development.' The preceding argument serves to establish another connection, between poverty in poor areas and public health in rich countries. The faraway poor are not enough of a nuisance and not enough of a threat for the rich of this world to goad the wealthy into collective action aimed at improving the lot of the indigent in remote areas. Yet, epidemics that are associated with poverty in other parts of the globe may one day provoke concerted action by the wealthy countries to eradicate the conditions of poverty that caused the spread of disease on a world scale.

The preceding argument was intended strictly as a thought experiment, serving to elucidate the dynamics that operate in the external effects of poverty and in the collective action required to fight it. A plague upon humanity is the last thing anyone should wish for. Rather one must hope that people, coordinated by states and international organizations, in time will find ways to overcome their dilemmas of collective action so as to lessen poverty and prevent epidemics in their global commune.

Note

1   An earlier version of this paper was presented as keynote speech at the Conference on Health and Social Change in the Integration of Europe, Budapest, August 1996.

Literature

Cipolla, C.M.
   1979   *I Pidocchi e il granduca; crisi economica e problemi sanitari nella Firenze del '600.* Bologna: Il Mulino.
De Swaan, A.
   1988   *In care of the state: Health care, education and welfare in Europe and the USA in the modern era.* Cambridge/New York: Polity Press/OUP.
Finer, S.E.
   1952   *The life and times of Sir Edwin Chadwick.* New York/London: Barnes & Noble/Methuen.
Garrett, L.
   1995   *The coming plague.* London: Penguin Books.

Gleichmann, P.R.

1979 'Städte reinigen und geruchlos machen: Menschliche Körperentleerungen, ihre Geräte und ihre Verhäuslichung.' In: H.Sturm (e d.), *Ästhetik und Umwelt.* Tübingen: Gunter Narr, pp. 99-132

Goubert, J.P.

1986 *La conquête de l'eau; l'avènement de la santé à l'âge industriel.* Paris: Laffont.

Kalff, E.

1995 *L'hygiénisation de la vie quotidienne: le logement insalubre à Paris (1830-1990)*, 2 vols., [diss. Université Paris vii].

Koolmees, P.A.

1997 *Symbolen van openbare hygiëne: Gemeentelijke slachthuizen in Nederland, 1795-1940.* [diss. Utrecht University] Rotterdam: Erasmus publishing.

La Berge, A.E.F.

1974 *Public health in France and the French public health movement, 1815-1848.* [diss. U. of Tennessee] Ann Arbor: University microfilms.

McCaa, Robert,

1996 'The big killers: Mortality crises in social context.' *Social Science History.* 20(4): 553-58.

McKeown, T.

1976 *The modern rise of population.* London: E. Arnold.

McNeill, W.H.

1976 *Plagues and peoples.* Garden City, ny: Doubleday.

Murard, L. & P. Zylberman

1985 'La raison de l'expert ou l'hygiène comme science sociale appliquée.' *Archives Européennes de sociologie* 26(1): 58-89.

Pelling, M.

1961 *Cholera, fever and English medicine, 1825-1865.* Cambridge: Harvard University Press.

Rosenberg, C.E.

1962 *The cholera years: the United States in 1832, 1849, and 1866.* Chicago and London: University of Chicago Press.

Rosenkrantz, B.G.

1972 *Public health and the state; changing views in Massachussets, 1842-1936.* Cambridge: Harvard University Press.

Van den Noort, J.

1990 *Pion of Pionier: Rotterdam – Gemeentelijke bedrijvigheid in de negentiende eeuw.* [diss. University of Leyden] Rotterdam: Historische publikaties Roterodamum.

Van der Heijden, C.G.W.P.

1994   'De Swaan getoetst. De aanleg en diffusie van het waterleidingstelsel in de industriestad Tilburg als collectief.' *Tijdschrift voor Sociale Geschiedenis* 20: 52-76.

1995a   *Het heeft niet willen groeien; Zuigelingen- en kindersterfte in Tilburg, 1820-1930; Omvang, oorzaken en maatschappelijkecontext.* Tilburg: St. zuidelijk historisch contact.

1995b   *Kleurloos, reukloos en smaakloos drinkwater: De watervoorziening in Tilburg vanaf het einde van de negentiende eeuw.* Tilburg: Tilburgse historische reeks.

Van Zon, H.

1986   *Een zeer onfrisse geschiedenis: Studies over niet-industriële vervuiling in Nederland, 1850-1920,* [diss. Groningen U.] Groningen.

Vigarello, G.

1985   *Le propre et le sale; l'hygiène du corps depuis le Moyen Age.* Paris: Éds. du Seuil.

CHAPTER III

Epidemics and Social Change

PIETER H. STREEFLAND

The expectation and occurrence of an epidemic are often accompanied by strong emotions, including fears of its dire consequences for people and their ways of life. Epidemics are also surrounded by uncertainty. One of the problems in preparing for and addressing the social effects of large-scale debilitating and often fatal disease is that there may not be sufficient knowledge about their content, direction and extent. It is not always clear what public policies and coping strategies would be appropriate to prepare for such an event. Prospective studies are needed, aiming at the description and analysis of the process of change as it unfolds. But what should such studies focus on? Our knowledge about the impact of epidemics on particular societies is obviously most extensive for those epidemics we have already survived. We appear to know far less, for example, about the social effects of the present-day AIDS pandemic instance, than about the effects of plague and cholera in the past.

In this contribution I shall first examine what is to be learned from the social history of some of the large epidemics of the past with respect to epidemic-induced social change. Research already done by historians of these upheavals may provide us with useful clues concerning what to look for in the present and anticipate for the future.

Social change is one of those broad concepts which requires limitation and specification. I shall include in the case studies examples of the often temporary social change which can occur when an epidemic prevails or is looming. A well-known one is the exacerbation of discrimination of minorities, who are held responsible for the disease and its devastation in some way. During the plague years in medieval Europe this fate struck the Jews, who were mercilessly prosecuted (Ziegler 1982). A more recent case, described by Kraut, is the collective aggression of Protestant Anglo-Saxon inhabitants of American cities against Irish immigrants at the time cholera reached these places in the first half of the 19th century (Kraut 1994).

In addition, I shall consider more lasting social effects of epidemics. A present day example that immediately comes to mind are the consequences that the AIDS epidemic has for rural households in many African countries. Due to the considerable mortality among the working age population, the implications of AIDS for livelihood support patterns and farming systems are disastrous (Barnett & Blaikie 1992).

To provide some depth to the discussion, I need to impose some restrictions on the subjects examined.[1] In regard to past epidemics, I want to focus on their socioeconomic effects, who is affected and how. Second, if applicable, I shall look specifically at the role and position of the state, at how it reacts and is responded to. Finally, I shall focus on epidemics of the infectious diseases plague and cholera in two regions with which I am most familiar: South Asia and Europe. Brief descriptions of the social consequences of plague and cholera, both of which still prevail in developing countries today, will be followed by a discussion of what a social science perspective of epidemics entails. The concepts imagined epidemic and social epidemic will be introduced. Next, building on the case material, I shall discuss essential research themes for prospective social science research on the social impact of epidemics. The contribution concludes with some remarks about new highly published epidemics.

Plague epidemics and social change

Medieval Europe

Plague epidemics have been particularly well researched and documented. Much is known, but we are always urged by historians to consider carefully, because there is also much uncertainty. Three aspects, which also have relevance to studies of other diseases, are especially important. One concerns figures; e.g. not all those labelled as plague victims actually died from plague, as causes of death could not be professionally verified, and especially deaths caused by famine were easily counted as plague victims.[2] Also, as David Arnold points out, true numbers were concealed at times 'in an attempt to evade intrusive state medical and sanitary measures' (1993: 202). In general, however, the numbers of those who died are appallingly high. The second aspect is that it is usually difficult to say whether an epidemic caused certain changes. As Ziegler remarks in regard to the Black Death in 14th century Europe, it 'did not initiate any major social or economic trend but it accelerated and modified – sometimes drastically – those that already existed.' (1982: 259) A third call for caution is expressed by Braudel (1967: 43) when he points out that accounts of past epidemics by contemporaries may describe signs and symptoms and use names of diseases which nowadays would be understood differently than at the time the observations were made. As I have only surveyed a small portion of the vast literature on the many plague epidemics that have prevailed, and there are differences in theoretical perspectives and interests of historians, combined with the temporal and geographic specificity of a plague epidemic, generalizations are not easy.

When describing the plague in late medieval Europe, Ziegler (1982) highlights the effects of that epidemic on the social fabric of rural society. The enormous death toll affected labour relations and labour conditions. The relations between landlords and tenants, the mobility of agricultural labourers, and the level of their wages changed considerably.

Another important observation is that the poor suffered the most from the disease, being most vulnerable. Ziegler also points out that the position of the clergy and the social organization of the church changed, at least temporarily. In addition, the religious beliefs and world view of the common people were modified by their terrifying experiences.

Nevertheless, the picture of how the plague affected, for instance, English rural society that Ziegler draws for us is one with considerable variety. Some of the changes that occurred did last, as was the case with enlargement of tenant holdings with land that had become free (1982: 263, 264). However, there was regional disparity and also a 'pattern... of losses made good, of a system strained but unbroken. Resilient and traditional, the manorial communities of England quickly put themselves back on an even keel and carried on, to the casual observer at least, as if the storm had never broken' (Ziegler 1982: 146).

Braudel, in his *Capitalism and Material Life 1400 – 1800*, stresses the migration of the rich from plague-stricken European towns: 'at the first sign of the disease the rich whenever possible took hurried flight to their country houses; no one thought of anything but himself...' (1973: 48). This flight often implied the disintegration of at least part of the municipal administrative and judicial apparatus. Urban life came largely to a standstill, with the poor remaining the sole inhabitants of the towns and main victims of the disease.

About effects of plague epidemics in 16th and 17th century Italy on the conditions of poor people and the way others perceived of the poor, Pullan writes that, as the poor were most usually the victims, they were often 'depicted as the means by which the whole social order was exposed to assault and depletion by fatal sickness, ...' (1995: 114). Consequently, they were objects of fear, as they were seen as 'the incubators and spreaders of disease, the gateway through which the plague might enter and fatally weaken society. But they were also a force for rebellion which might well take possession of the half-deserted towns from which their masters had fled' (1995: 106, 107).

However, the disease also brought more work for the poor, especially for the vagrants and criminals among them, to carry out essential services as cleaning and undertaking. Also, in order to protect their populations, those out of work or quarantined in their houses received food support from municipalities using public funds. It leads Pullan to conclude that in urban Italy the poor had three contrasting roles, that of bearers, victims, and beneficiaries of the plague (1995: 107). Slack, referring to the wider European context, also mentions how the epidemics led to a sharper etching of the dichotomy between the rich and the poor in the towns, particularly since the former considered the latter 'with the contempt of the respectable for the masses who presented a threat to their health, their social position, and their peace of mind' (1988: 448).

Finally, Slack (1988) emphasizes the contribution of plague epidemics to state formation by way of strengthening local urban government institutions regulating the behaviour of both those suffering from plague and the, still, healthy. Watts (1997: 16) highlights both the benevolent and the restrictive aspects of such plague regulation, when he summarizes Italian plague-control in five elements: rigorous policing of human movement by way of quarantine, compulsory burial of plague deaths and destruction of their possessions, isolation of the sick and their families, provision of free medical service and food to the isolated, and provision of subsistence to the poor. He then continues to describe how people resented the tough regime, grumbled about it but, subsequently, adjusted their ways of life.

British India around the turn of the century

Moving now to the South, I shall describe some of the ways in which the plague has affected Indian society. The focus is, first, on the epidemic that prevailed around the turn of the present century when India was still a colony and included the present countries of India, Pakistan and Bangladesh. In his book *Plagues and Peoples*, William McNeill (1979: 148) points out how the spreading of this global epidemic of bubonic plague was related to the emergence of a steamship network. Before that 'in the days of sail, the oceans had simply been too wide for the disease to survive on shipboard long enough to make a lodgment in the seaports and waiting rodent communities of America and South Africa. But when steamships began to travel faster and, being bigger, perhaps also carried larger populations of rats among whom the infection could circulate longer, the oceans suddenly became permeable as never before.' He continues to mention that in several places 'infected ships, rats and their fleas ... managed to infect their wild cousins ...' According to Ian Catanach (1983) this is exactly what happened in India: the plague reached India in 1896 by steamship from Hong Kong; from Bombay plague-stricken rats and fleas spread it throughout India. He also mentions the important role of a local rodent, the gerbil, in this process of spreading the disease. He highlights that in India, plague was to a large extent an urban epidemic, except in the Punjab, where it mainly prevailed in the villages, which according to Catanach could be explained by the specific role of the gerbil. In the Punjabi villages the incidence of plague led to extensive migration, but it also caused an interruption of some of the migratory patterns prevailing before. The new migration pattern was often rather localized as people fled to nearby places where they had kinship and marriage relations. An interesting observation is that the Muslims tended to stay in their own village, as their religious teaching told them not to flee from God's will and justice. The discontinuation of old migration patterns mainly concerned seasonal immigration by agricultural labourers from other districts, who avoided plague-stricken areas.

Another issue pursued by Catanach (1988: 2, 3) is one that social historians, as we saw earlier, have researched in depth for the plague in Europe: Were the rich or the poor affected most? Catenach makes an interesting observation about this in relation to the Indian plague as it developed in Bombay. He states that in the early outbreaks the wealthier inhabitants appear to have suffered the most, but that as plague spread over the city and the more well-to-do fled, it was specifically the poor that appeared to be hit worst. According to him, much remains unclear regarding this theme. Another historian, Ira Klein (1986) does, however, emphasize that plague did, indeed, tend to appear in the poor areas of Bombay. What we should remember is Catanach's indication of how the epidemic evolved. The social effects, including differential mortality among the social classes, are related to the manner in which the epidemic develops, to the epidemic as a process. He also stressed this process character of the epidemic in his discussions of plague in the rural Punjab, indicating that although plague remained there for many years, it did not strike with the same severity every year and not yearly in the same village (1988: 4). There is, in other words, variety and disparity, as we also saw in Ziegler's description of the events in medieval England.

Arnold (1993) and Chandavarkar (1995) situate the plague epidemic in the larger political arena, namely that of the colonial state. They describe how the state intervened much more in the daily life of people than before, in the case of other epidemics, in particular those of smallpox and cholera. Chandavarkar writes that the 'forceful and aggressive intrusion of the colonial state into the private domain was not simply dramatic and brutal but also novel and unprecedented' (1995: 208). Both authors describe how slum dwellings were destroyed, houses and their inhabitants examined in military-style detection operations (Chandavarkar's term), train passengers inspected and people quarantined. Indeed, the very important local sensitivities regarding caste behavioral rules or convictions on the segregation of men and women were largely ignored. Not surprisingly, such measures led to strong opposition, both in the local Indian press and through demonstrations, rumours and emergence of new beliefs regarding the legitimacy of colonial rule. Such opposition was not without effect: 'from 1898 to 1900 plague measures in most provinces of India were liberalised as a result of suspicion and hostility among lower-class Indians; and, on a local level, medical officers and administrators began to enter into a dialogue with community leaders about how best to conduct measures against plague' (Harrison 1994: 146).

The plague epidemic affected not only the relationships between colonial rulers and Indians. As it easily crossed social and national borders, it also had important implications for the international economic and political relations of Britain and British India. Harrison, in his *Public Health in British India*, highlights how 'in the first weeks, the authorities in Bombay did their best to reassure the populace and the international community that the disease was not true plague, but "bubonic fever" or "plague of a mild type"' (1994: 133). Soon, however, the existence of full-blown plague was admitted, and 'indeed, within a few days quarantine had been imposed against Indian vessels at Suez and at numerous ports around the world, with varying degrees of severity' (1994: 134). Besides, the government was forced to impose full quarantine against major Indian harbours like Madras, Calcutta and Karachi (1994: 134). As a consequence of such measures, together with a very substantial emigration, Bombay broke down totally as a commercial center. Not only the commercial impact of the quarantine was important, it also meant a restrictive effect on the international pilgrimage of Muslims. Harrison explains how this not only led to tensions within the imperial order, but also to strains between Hindu and Muslim leadership in India (1994: 136, 137).

The plague in Surat in 1994

We now jump forward in time to the plague epidemic that struck in Surat, Western India, in late 1994. The Indian sociologist Ganshyam Shah made a study of the social implications of this epidemic (Shah 1997). His perspective is that of the political economy of disease, relating the epidemic to the poor conditions of the public health system in the fast growing town of Surat, where seasonal epidemics of infectious diseases like malaria and diarrhoea are a normal occurrence. He emphasizes that this urban epidemic of pneumonic plague was localized and brief: between mid-September and Mid-October 1994. He also mentions the relatively low mortality: less than a hundred people died.

Not surprisingly, when Shah makes statements on the social and political consequences of the Surat plague, his comparative frame of reference is that of the plague epidemic in British India discussed above, which killed millions and lasted for two decades.[3] He points out that since then, people's ideas and behaviour in regard to caste differences, purity and pollution have changed and weakened, as have their, at times related, attitudes to Western medicine and hospitals. In other words, not only did the characteristics of the epidemics differ, but also the social, cultural and political contexts within which they occurred had drastically changed.

Regarding the socioeconomic groups most heavily hit by the epidemic, he concludes that these were factory workers and casual labourers. By far, most of the victims were male, which may be related to the fact that many were migrants, who had left their families in the home village. Many people fled the town, but among them the more well-to-do seem to have been over-represented. Referring to a survey by the Surat Municipal Corporation during the early days of the plague, Shah tells that nearly one third of the houses of Surat were deserted, most of the inhabitants presumably having fled (1994: 152-162). Medical practitioners were the first to flee the city, closing their dispensaries. They were followed by industrial entrepreneurs and businessmen, and in due course a real exodus took place, leaving a city inhabited to a much larger extent than before by the elderly, the disabled and the poor. In his account Shah also emphasizes the important work of those doctors and civil servants who remained behind and fulfilled their responsibilities. There was a lot of fear and rumours, leading to all kinds of avoidance and protest behaviour, not only in Surat, but all over India. And also beyond India; in fact, all over the world.

In fact, what developed in India in 1994 was a small localized epidemic with enormous global reverberations. It was, however, not so much the biomedically defined epidemic (the actual epidemiological characteristics of the disease, including numbers affected, organism responsible and pattern of transmission) that mattered. Although dangerous and deadly, the disease was not extremely virulent and was soon under control with the use of antibiotics – a superior medical technology which had, of course, not been available a hundred years earlier. The epidemiological surveillance apparatus was in place, even though it reacted slowly in the early stages of the epidemic. It was the *imagined epidemic* that mattered, including the fear of presently unknown but vaguely heard of pandemics, fears that had recently been kindled by the emergence of AIDS, supposedly killing thousands, if not millions in Africa. It became clear that somewhere in the collective consciousness, some memories lingered, notions about the disaster of large-scale and deadly contagious disease.[4,5]

There were clear global shock waves. Tourists decided to avoid India, and trade from that country was temporarily suspended. Planes and ships from the country were handled with care. In India the epidemic and the imagined epidemic became the subjects of political discussion on the negligence of the civil service in handling urban growth and decay. Once medical control was established and large-scale fatalities did not occur, when public confidence had returned and the parameters of the epidemic became clearer and accepted by the general population, then the imagined epidemic evaporated, both in India and abroad, although much damage had been done. Trade had suffered greatly, and once more India, strongly aspiring to the status and external image of a modern nation state, had been identified with disease, dirtiness and a stumbling government apparatus.

It is important to remind ourselves that also the earlier and much larger epidemics in the nineteenth and early twentieth centuries had important international ramifications. In the second half of the last century, there were several international meetings which aimed at setting regulations to curtail the spreading of plague and what was called at the time 'Asiatic cholera'. One such conference, held in Constantinople in 1866 declared pilgrimage gatherings in India one of the main epidemic sources of cholera (Arnold 1993: 186). At another one, held in Venice in 1897, the threat of the plague was discussed, and the British colonial administration was pressured to take measures resulting, for instance, in curtailing the Hajj, the pilgrimage to

Mecca (Arnold 1993: 205). McNeill (1979: 254, 255) also points at this international cooperation and how it resulted in new regulations for health and international travel when at the end of the last century the smallpox vaccination became available.

There are, however, important differences between the global ramifications of present-day epidemics and those of the past. The earlier international discussions and formulation of regulations concerned interactions and negotiations between states. To a much larger extent than is the case nowadays, changes in international trade and in people's mobility which were induced by epidemics followed by curtailing actions of states. In the case of the Surat plague and of other contemporary localized epidemics of (re)emerging diseases, there may be advice forthcoming from the state or from the medical profession, but essentially it is people themselves and commercial companies (airlines) who take avoidance or curtailing decisions. Global mobility appears to have been liberalized considerably as long as the scope of epidemic threat is limited (see also contribution De Swaan, this volume).

Cholera epidemics and social change

Cholera in British India

In Eastern India, particularly in Bengal, cholera was, and is, an endemic disease that occasionally spread(s) in an epidemic form to other parts of the subcontinent. It strikes suddenly and randomly, with appalling symptoms – cramps, severe vomiting and diarrhoea, shivering, sweating, a deadly pallor – and kills swiftly (Arnold 1993: 160; McNeill 1979: 240). It was considered a terrifying and exceptionally destructive disease by both the Indians and the British (Arnold 1993: 159).

In 1817 'epidemic' cholera, which was perceived as a new disease by the British colonial soldiers, citizens, administrators and medical professionals, spread outside Eastern India, initially to other parts of the subcontinent, but in due course to the Middle East and Europe. The disease 'made a profound impression on Europeans, arousing more fear and interest than any other disease... No disease was more important, and no disease as little understood, as "epidemic cholera"' (Harrison 1994: 99). This image is completed by the description of Arnold who emphasizes the political character of cholera, by mentioning how it challenged British colonial power, and its role in exacerbating social divisions, for instance those within colonial society between rulers and subjects (1993: 159). He points out how Indian rituals to propitiate the disease, ranging from the sacrifice of a buffalo to the expulsion of an outcaste from the village or the circulation of earthen pots from village to village, to the British 'were a reminder of the great cultural gulf that divided the colonizers from the colonized and drew attention to the existence of patterns of rural solidarity and lateral communication over which the state had little control' (1993: 178).

The various cholera epidemics which affected the society of British India had the following more specific social effects. Among the Indian population the disease struck the poor most violently, particularly those living in the urban slums of Calcutta, Bombay and Madras (Arnold 1993: 166). The coincidence of the cholera epidemic of 1856-57 with the Mutiny of 1857 (the most important uprising against British rule in India in the last century) severely curtailed the effectiveness of the British troops in quelling the insurrection (Harrison 1994: 61). The linkage of cholera epidemics and of the spreading of that disease with Hindu pilgrimage and pilgrimage centers such as Puri and Hardwar led to pressure on the British by other governments to take curtailing measures. The British colonial administration, fearing more unrest after the Mutiny, refused to do so, but their investigations of the matter and reference to it in literature and press put another strain on the relation between the colonial state and the Indians it ruled.[6]

Cholera in Europe

Despite the international efforts to prevent it, in 1831 cholera arrived from Asia in Europe. Both De Swaan (1990) and Evans (1990, 1995), when writing on the effects of cholera there, stress the feelings of terror and shock which accompanied its arrival in urban society. Evans concludes that statistics suggest that although cholera 'could and did affect the well-off and the rich, its impact on the poor was disproportionately high in most epidemics' (1995: 155-157). This impact included both greater incidence of the disease and a higher proportion of deaths. The rich could flee, their occupations did not bring them into contact with contaminated water, they could also live more hygienically, and their better nutritional status improved their survival chances if they became infected (Evans 1992). From Evans'(1990) detailed study of the effects of cholera in the city of Hamburg between 1830 and 1910, we learn that there was differentiation in levels of vulnerability and coping capacity among the poor, which might be related to differences in the households' dependencies and patronage relations with the church or a benevolent employer.

The objective picture of the poor being hit the hardest by cholera was also the subjective view of the well-to-do. They saw the disease as carried and spread by the poor, blaming them for their filthy way of life, and sometimes seeing it as God's punishment for their sins.

The association between poverty, squalor and cholera in the prevailing moral, political and scientific discourse in 19th century urban Europe is a major point of departure of De Swaan when he develops his ideas on the emergence of collective sanitary arrangements (De Swaan 1990: 124-142; also his contribution in this volume). He puts the most emphasis on the rising awareness of the interdependence of all urban inhabitants and the need to collectively do something about this. Ultimately, during a process in which a pragmatic elite of doctors, teachers and engineers formed a vanguard, this encouraged the rise of and public support for the realization of public sanitation measures.

The mid-19th century was a volatile period in European political history, and not surprisingly Evans (1995) also pursues the question of what role cholera played in the nineteenth century revolutionary uprisings, pointing, like others before him, at the coincidence of epidemics and revolution, as was the case in 1848. He shows that cholera was a cause of social unrest among the poor, who blamed the authorities and particularly the medical profession for killing off their class by introducing or furthering the disease. But a definite link between the incidence of cholera epidemics and wider politically inspired upheavals has not been established.

Imagined and social epidemics

This succinct exercise in retrospective learning reveals that epidemics have completely different meanings from different perspectives. Though some perspectives, like that of the victim or the medical professional, appear constant in any situation, all are coloured by specific historical and cultural conditions. Nevertheless, it is useful to differentiate between epidemics on the basis of the perspective from which they are perceived or defined by people, groups or organizations.

Nowadays, the biomedical perspective of an epidemic is foremost that of the epidemiologists. They define its immediate causes, mode of transmission, populations at risk, natural history of the disease and ways of controlling it.[7]

However, their views represent, to the extent that they are made public, only one of the bits of information that shape the public views and expectations of an epidemic. In the case of the recent plague in Surat, we saw that people's reactions were shaped by the medical manifestations of the outbreak (acute disease and death), the information provided by public health professionals and through the media, and prevailing memories, ideas and emotions. On the basis of all this, the *imagined epidemic* emerged. The collective flight, which certainly hampered efforts to control the outbreak, was a clear consequence of the imagined epidemic, as was the temporary avoidance of India by tourists.

There are two aspects of an imagined epidemic that I wish to emphasize here. First, it is a manifestation of what sociologists call the Thomas theorem: 'if men define situations as real, they are real in their consequences' (Merton 1967: 421), which Merton later developed into his theory of the self-fulfilling prophecy. An interesting contemporary example of the development and implications of an imagined epidemic is, of course, BSE or mad cow's disease and the related CJD (Creutzfeld Jacob Disease) epidemic among humans. Here we see that people change their dietary habits because of the combination of the expected consequences of eating contaminated meat and a lack of trust in the civil authorities and politicians who assure them that it is now safe to eat meat. In general, one could say that the Thomas theorem has a high applicability value in the case of epidemics. The pervading atmosphere of uncertainty and anxiety creates conditions in which people take collective decisions based not on fact, but on particular interpretations, setting in motion a train of events.

Second, imagined epidemics are constructed on the basis of many sources. They include actual experiences of acute and virulent disease in many people, which possibly resulted in death. They also embody memories of and stories about past epidemics, bits of biomedical information, rumours that are impossible to check, and news stories. As these points of reference differ between and within populations, it is possible to find narratives about rather different imagined epidemics which refer to the same actual outbreak. Accordingly, imagined epidemics of victims, potential victims, survivors, civil administrators, national and international public health officials and media reporters may emerge, as different versions of the same plague.[8] Nevertheless, there is also considerable overlap, forming the basis for collective reactions such as flight, avoidance, control measures and resistance against such regulation and restraint.

In addition to the imagined epidemic, which is very much an emic or insider's phenomenon, it is also useful to distinguish a *social epidemic*. This is the non-medical professional outsider's definition or representation of an epidemic, including its social impact, its social and behavioural causes and ways of spreading. The representations and interpretations of the social historians presented earlier in this paper, based on documents, biographies, fiction and sometimes oral history, are examples of such social epidemics. So are the views and findings of sociologists and anthropologists studying new outbreaks.

Accordingly, the Surat outbreak of plague was epidemiologically defined as a local outbreak, but sociologically as rooted in urban poverty and socio-economic differentiation and resulting in national and global social and economic consequences. Apart from all that, however, imagined epidemics developed in the minds of people in Surat itself, elsewhere in India and even beyond, leading some of them to flee the city and others not to visit India for a while.

When discussing the plague in Europe and British India, we saw that it is important to consider the process of an epidemic. The disease may initially affect the rich and move to the poor, or start with the poor and never infect the rich because they flee. It may be urban initially and then spread to rural areas, or remain an urban phenomenon throughout its course. It may last decades, or be over swiftly. It may have long latent periods, as in the case of AIDS and BSE related CJD. It may be fatal or lead to disablement or, as was the case with smallpox, disfigurement.

The epidemic as a process refers to more than how the disease manifests itself, who are affected and in what way. It also concerns developments in perceptions and reactions. Rosenberg (1992: 278-287) has approached this process character of an epidemic by using the metaphor of a drama. Accordingly, he distinguishes the dramatic acts of progressive revelation (the epidemic is recognized as such), managing randomness (collective explanations originate), negotiating public response (collective reactions and rituals appear), and subsidence and retrospection (the evaluation of policy makers and historians). It is particularly in the second stage that the collective interpretations emerge and the imagined epidemics are constructed. They are not stationary, however, but evolve.

In his introduction to the important collection of essays *Epidemics and Ideas*, Paul Slack summarizes that the most radical responses occur among the population affected by an epidemic which is novel, violent and intense, and random, or at least perceived as such (Slack 1995: 7). In the same volume Richard Evans, when trying to relate the European cholera epidemics to the 1830 and 1848 revolutions, points out that really very high levels of mortality are required for a profound level of social impact (Evans 1995: 170).

Elsewhere, Slack (1988) emphasizes another theme, namely that the regular incidence of epidemics of the same disease (plague) over a longer period enhance the predictability of the disease and, hence, the possibility for social responses to become institutionalized.

Interesting and important observations like these could be fitted into a theoretical framework to explain the characteristics and course of imagined and social epidemics. Such a framework would be a valuable addition to epidemiological theories about epidemics (cf. Anderson & May 1991).

Themes of change

I shall now continue with the discussion of themes which are important for research into social and imagined epidemics. Earlier elements of these themes of change were described in specific social, political, temporal and geographic contexts. Another source is the explanatory framework outlined in the last section. A few themes which received less emphasis in the earlier descriptive sections, although they are certainly important, will also be mentioned.

The first research theme is that of the role and position of the state at the time of epidemics. How do epidemics affect the state? Do they result in its strengthening or lead to or exacerbate its disintegration and decline? Of course, the contrasting question of how the disintegration of states induces epidemics is also extremely relevant. We only have to think about the increased chances of epidemics of immunizable diseases when government health care breaks down.

What became clear in various cases was that epidemics demand that the state, or the local administration, take a position. Epidemic outbreaks are pre-eminently occasions for the state to assert its authority and act in protection of its citizens. In certain cases, like colonial situations, the state is inclined to represent the interests of different classes of citizens in a differential manner. Nevertheless, the emotions surrounding epidemics, as well as the medical interpretations, require equity in the state's treatment of different groups, and perceived dismeanour will be forcefully reacted to. In the case of cholera in Europe, it became clear that an epidemic and the collective requirements to control it may contribute to the process of state formation. In relation to plague in European towns, the strengthening of the local administration in the process of carrying out new, epidemic-induced tasks has been mentioned.

Then there are the significant popular reactions to an epidemic. This theme needs to be studied at different levels of social integration. At the level of individuals, it involves coping with uncertainty, anxiety, fear and suffering. At the level of families and households, it involves coping with disease, death, loss of income and disintegration, At levels of communities and kinship networks, the epidemic affects mutual support patterns. If epidemics recur over a longer period, ways of coping may solidify into cultural patterns. Popular reactions also include uprisings and demonstrations; accusations and rumours; new religious explanations. When studying popular reactions we need to understand the imagined epidemics. Hence our research would need to include the form and contents of different kinds of narratives about the epidemic, with attention being paid to the metaphors and images used.

A third theme of social change is how an epidemic affects the structural aspects of society. This includes issues like the breakdown of mutual support patterns; changes in leadership patterns; the form of migration caused by the epidemic; how labour relations are affected; and gender relations. This also covers implications for civil society: for the churches, various kinds of associations, political parties.

An epidemic's consequences for livelihood support systems, such as farming systems and the realm of small businesses, supplies the next major theme. We know that disease often has cumulative effects for the survival of households, as income deteriorates and costs of medical treatment form an additional burden. In this way an epidemic can have a devastating effect on the economic basis of villages and urban quarters. Due to their susceptibility and vulnerability and lack of sufficient coping capacity, it is the poor who are generally affected the most and the most seriously by an epidemic. Studies on livelihood effects should, therefore, focus primarily on them.[9]

A fifth theme to be mentioned here involves the demographic consequences. How are the population's age structure, dependency ratios, and fertility affected? Finally, the last theme concerns the effects of an epidemic on medical discourse, in general as well as on public health policy, and on the role of physicians.

Concluding remarks

With the clear exception of the AIDS pandemic, present-day epidemics appear to be different from those of cholera and plague described in this contribution. They usually affect smaller populations and certainly kill fewer people. Although some of them are extremely virulent, like Ebola and Lassa fever, they also sound rather exotic to those who live in the North. It seems as if such outbreaks belong to the South and cannot easily reach people who live in the North, since they are protected by an epidemiological surveillance apparatus and a public health system that are securely in place. Yet the unexpected arrival of HIV and AIDS in the 1980s, and the current re-emergence of tuberculosis in Northern countries teach us that, wherever we live, deadly epidemics are an intrinsic part of our world. In fact, with increased global travel and trade and the persistence of poverty and deficient health care systems, the chances of outbreaks of infectious disease have certainly not decreased (see Kager, this volume).

In addition, a new class of non-infectious disease epidemics in the North appears to have emerged, vaguely defined and related to life and working styles; for example, ME (myalgic encephalomyelitis), leading to a condition of chronic and extreme tiredness, or repetitive strain injuries (RSI), associated with prolonged computer keyboard use and a wrong body posture, leading to incapacity of joints and muscles. BSE related CJD should, possibly, also be included. There appears to be more that we don't know about the natural history of such diseases and about their effects on society than we do know. We have a great deal of information on these diseases, which fuels our imagination but does not systematically contribute to our knowledge about their possible social consequences, how to avert them and how to prepare ourselves to face them. It is important that we are alert to the social implications long before they occur on a large scale.

All epidemics are also social and imagined epidemics. People react to their occurrence on the basis of their interpretations. The diseases influence the lives and the patterns of living together of those involved, often drastically, leading to new social and cultural adjustments. Much, not all, social change caused by epidemics is detrimental.

In this contribution I gave an impression of the wide range of social change that epidemics can lead to. I emphasized the importance for prospective research into such change in the case of new epidemics. To guide such studies, we need a set of major research themes, a number of which have been elaborated.

Notes

1 Due to these restrictions, some major themes have to be left out. One important example involves the consequences which particularly McNeill (1979) stresses epidemics have had in the political arena at the time of invasions and conquests,

for instance, in regard to the 'great dying' which the arrival of conquering Spaniards and Portuguese brought to the Americas (Wolf 1982: 133). It may appear that this could not so easily happen nowadays, but just imagine that AIDS had come to Southeast Asia not in the late 1980s but 25 years earlier. How would that have affected the willingness of the American population to send their young sons and husbands to the Vietnam War and to their spells of rest and recreation in Manila and Bangkok?

2 Still, the statement of the 1920 Sialkot District Gazetteer, composed under British Indian colonial rule, that 'on one occasion a man who died from the results of breaking his leg was reported to have died of plague' is probably one of the exceptions in this regard.

3 Shah (1997: 222) notes that the enormous difference in mortality between the epidemics appears to have been related to the relatively low degree of virulence of the 1994 organism spreading the disease.

4 Such fears can, sometimes, also be recognized in language. A clear example involves some Dutch expressions used to curse someone, such as 'krijg the pest' (catch the plague), 'tyfuslijer' (typhus patient) and 'krijg de kolere' (catch the cholera) or more general expressions, like 'de pest ergens over in hebben' (being mad at something, freely translated: being angry about something as if it was the plague) of 'ergens een pesthekel aan hebben' (to hate something like the plague).

5 In Surat, according to Shah (1997: 151), it was only exceptional individuals who held some fading memories of an earlier plague epidemic. 'As in Europe, there was no collective memory of the destruction by plague. All they new was that it was a dangerous disease.'

6 In British India cholera was defined as a specific Indian disease to which the scientific discussions regarding cholera which took place in the second half of the nineteenth century in Europe were not really relevant. This assumption played according to Harrison (1996) an important role in determining government policy in the colony.

7 Though there still may be different medical interpretations about certain parameters of specific epidemics, such differences used to be much more striking and visible in the past. De Swaan, in his contribution to this volume, discusses the differences between adherents of the miasmatic view and contagionists in explaining the causes and mode of transmission of cholera in the last century.

8 It is important to understand that biomedical representations of an epidemic and the concomitant views of civil administrators, politicians and public health officials are shaped in a sociocultural context, including political stresses, associations with past disasters, and fears of being too late, doing too little. A good example is that of the swine flu epidemic that never really was, except as an imagined epidemic. Still, in 1976 in the USA a decision was taken to spend US$ 135 million of federal money to develop and implement a large scale vaccination programme (Garrett 1995, Ch. 6).

9 Farmer (1996) rightly emphasizes the importance of positioning the study of (re)emerging diseases in a framework of social inequality.

Literature

Anderson, R.M. & R.M. May

1991   *Infectious diseases of humans: Dynamics and control.* Oxford: OUP.

Arnold, D.

1993   *Colonizing the body: State medicine and epidemic disease in nineteenth century India.* Berkeley: University of California Press.

Barnett, T. & P. Blaikie

1992   *AIDS in Africa: Its present and future impact. London: Belhaven Press.*

Braudel, F.

1973   *Capitalism and material life 1400-1800.* London: Weidenfeld and Nicholson.

Catanach, I.J.

1983   'Plague and the Indian village, 1896-1914.' In: P.G. Robb (ed.), *Rural India: Land, power and society under British rule.* London: Curzon Press, pp. 216-244.

1988   *Some demographic aspects of plague in India, 1896-1916.* Position paper for the Third World Economic History Group, SOAS, 31 May 1988, 8 pp.

Chandavarkar, R.

1995   'Plague panic and epidemic politics in India, 1896-1914.' In: T. Ranger & P. Slack (eds), *Epidemics and ideas.* Paperback edition. Cambridge: Cambridge University Press, pp. 101-125.

De Swaan, A.

1990   *In care of the state: health care, education and welfare in Europe and the USA in the modern era.* Paperback edition. Cambridge: Polity Press.

Evans, R.J.

1990   *Death in Hamburg: Society and politics in the cholera years 1830-1910.* Harmondsworth: Penguin Books.

1995   'Epidemics and revolutions: Cholera in nineteenth century Europe.' In: T. Ranger & P. Slack (eds), *Epidemics and ideas.* Paperback edition. Cambridge: Cambridge University Press, pp. 149-175.

Farmer, P.

1996   'Social inequalities and emerging infectious diseases.' *Emerging Infectious Diseases* 2(4): 259-270.

Garrett, L.

1995   *The coming plague: Newly emerging diseases in a world out of balance.* Harmondsworth: Penguin Books.

Gazetteer of the Sialkot District 1920
    1921   'Lahore: Superintendent government printing.' Reprinted 1990. Lahore:
            Sangemeel Publication.
Harrison, M.
    1994   *Public health in British India.* Cambridge: Cambridge University Press.
    1996   'A question of locality: The identity of cholera in British India, 1860-1890.'
            In: D. Arnold (ed.), *Warm climates and western medicine.* Editions Rodopi:
            Amsterdam, pp. 133-160.
Klein, I.
    1986   'Urban development and death: Bombay city, 1870-1914.' *Modern Asian
            Studies* 20: 725-54.
Knaus, A.M.
    1994   *Silent travellers: Germs, genes, and the 'immigrant menace'.* Baltimore:
            Johns Hopkins University Press.
Merton, R.K.
    1967   *Social theory and social structure.* 12th printing. New York: The Free
            Press.
McNeill, W.H.
    1979   *Plagues and peoples.* Harmondsworth: Penguin Books.
Pullan, B.
    1995   'Plague and perceptions of the poor in early modern Italy.' In: T. Ranger
            & P. Slack (eds), *Epidemics and ideas.* Paperback edition. Cambridge:
            Cambridge University Press, pp. 101-125.
Rosenberg, C.E.
    1992   *Explaining epidemics and other studies in the history of medicine.* Cam-
            bridge: Cambridge University Press.
Shah, G.
    1997   *Public health and urban development: The plague in Surat.* New Delhi:
            Sage.
Slack, P.
    1988   'Responses to plague in early medieval Europe: The implications of public
            health.' *Social Research* 55(3): 433-454.
    1995   'Introduction.' In: T. Ranger & P. Slack (eds.), *Epidemics and ideas.* Paper-
            back edition. Cambridge: Cambridge University Press, pp. 1-21.
Watts, S.
    1997   *Epidemics and history: Disease, power and imperialism.* New Haven: Yale
            University Press.
Wolf, E.R.
    1982   *Europe and the people without history.* Berkeley: University of California
            Press.
Ziegler, P.
    1982   *The black death.* Reprinted. Harmondsworth: Penguin Books.

CHAPTER IV

Social Sciences and Aids:
New Fields, New Approaches

CORLIEN M. VARKEVISSER

When in the early 1980s it became clear that mankind was confronted with a new disease AIDS, caused by a virus that appeared to be extremely difficult to control, the first reaction in the Western world was disbelief and panic. Both the medical profession and the general public were shocked by increasingly alarming news: an ever greater proportion of the infected persons appeared to be dying, while the prospects of developing cures or vaccines in the near future were dim. Though knowledge of the routes and rate of transmission increased rapidly, many unanswered questions remained.

Medical professionals had to face the potential risk they ran by treating patients who might be HIV-infected. In the Netherlands, dentists started wearing masks in those days. Incidents of doctors refusing to operate on patients known to be HIV infected hit the news. Health policy makers were confronted with the ethical dilemma of how to reconcile an HIV-infected person's rights to confidentiality with the public interest of protecting the population from infection. Some countries, e.g. China and the USA, made it obligatory for foreigners to provide a medical certificate of being HIV-free before they would be permitted to enter the country.[1]

In developing countries the first reactions were disbelief and denial. Here disbelief did not relate so much to the unexpected failure of the medical profession to control the new disease as to the estimated magnitude of the problem and the risk of being infected. Unlike the situation in the USA and Western Europe, where during the first years of the epidemic, transmission of HIV limited itself to homosexual males and injecting drug users, in the South the major route of infection was unprotected heterosexual behaviour, followed by transmission from mother to child, and contact with HIV-infected blood through unsterile injections or unscreened blood transfusions.[2] This implied that virtually the entire population was at risk. The intense concern of the medical profession at global level initially met with slow response and sometimes was just ignored among policy makers and the population (Barnett & Blaikie 1992; Caldwell et al. 1992; Meursing 1997).

This reaction is understandable. In regions where disease and death are still common in all age groups (Kager, this volume) and where economic crises, droughts and political unrest compete for attention, the appearance of a new disease, whose massive mortality has not yet been demonstrated, is just one of many concerns. The long time it takes before HIV-infected persons develop visible symptoms, and the unfamiliarity with the link between the weakening of a seropositive's immune system and the occurrence of commonly known diseases, such as tuberculosis or chronic diarrhoea, masked the increasing prevalence of HIV infection. Moreover, since HIV, like other sexually transmitted diseases (STDs), often carries connotations of shame and stigma, even if patients and their relatives suspected HIV infection, they would not easily discuss the matter. A large proportion of HIV infection is not diagnosable, because in sub-Saharan Africa the possibilities for HIV testing and the health staff's knowledge of AIDS are limited (Todd & Barongo 1997). And if there is proof that someone is HIV positive, the health workers are often reluctant to convey the bad news to the patient. For all these reasons AIDS was and still is, to a large extent, surrounded by silence (cf. Meursing 1997).

Another factor creating disbelief and even distrust in the South was the cultural background of those who reported the growing epidemic and stressed the need for changes in sexual behaviour. These messengers were predominantly white, or at least associated with Western culture. Local newspapers expressed doubt whether AIDS existed, or indeed spread as rapidly as official, international sources suggested.[3] In Eastern Africa the rumour circulated that 'the Americans' were purposively infecting the African continent with AIDS through condoms which, instead of preventing HIV transmission, transmitted the virus (Pool et al. 1995; Mwizarubi et al. 1997). Western jealousy about the potency of African people was purported to be one of the motives.

Such accusative rumours are common in times of uncontrollable epidemic stress and have been reported throughout history in different parts of the world (Streefland, this volume). Accordingly, in the USA, the AIDS epidemic provoked suspicions that immigrants from Haiti had introduced the virus, whereas research suggested it was more likely that HIV had spread in the reverse direction (Farmer 1992). The Western press prematurely pointed at Zaire and Central Africa as the cradle of the disease, which led to emotional reactions in Africa.

Doubts about the seriousness of the epidemic have been overtaken by history. Within 15 years, the scattered outbreaks of AIDS throughout the Americas, Europe and sub-Saharan Africa have spread like wild fire. By the end of 1995, 21 million adults and 1.5 million children were estimated to be affected, of whom 16 million reside in sub-Saharan Africa. Over 5 million had died. The disease is spreading by roughly 10,000 new infections a day. In 1996 it was assumed that by the year 2000 there will be over 30 million affected cases (Quinn 1996).[4]

Such global trends mask differences within continents and countries. The first signs of stabilization of the disease in sub-Saharan Africa, to which this contribution particularly refers, stem from areas where the epidemic was first reported: Uganda and surrounding countries (Madraa & Ruranga-Rubaramira 1996; Mulder et al. 1995). Rates of infection in these areas remain high, however, and the further course of the epidemic is still unknown.

The rapid increase of the disease appears to be determined by a number of closely interrelated factors including poverty, mobility of the population, political instability, risky sexual behaviour within rapidly changing socio-cultural contexts, and poorly functioning health care systems. All these factors prove difficult to influence. As yet, prospects for control of the disease are dim. Development of a vaccine is still a distant promise. The multidrug regimen newly available in the North is extremely demanding on the patient's cooperation, while its costs are prohibitive for developing countries, and the long-term results are still dubious due to emerging drug resistance. Safe sexual behaviour is therefore at present still the major device to cut the transmission of HIV.

Questions and attempts at responses

A new, rapidly spreading deadly infectious disease like AIDS poses many challenges to scientists and policy makers. First, questions and uncertainties exist with regard to the parameters of the epidemic: the (increasing) magnitude and distribution of infection, the causes and risk factors in transmission, the clinical manifestations and progression of the disease. Second, the challenges concern possibilities for control. The socio-economic and emotional consequences of the disease for the infected, their families and communities, for the health services and the society at large, and the way in which all concerned cope with these consequences form the third category of problems.

From the beginning it was clear that different scientific disciplines had to unite forces in order to find answers. The social sciences would have to play their part in describing and interpreting the wide spectrum of responses to the pandemic. A major question for social scientists was to provide insight into the various forms and determinants of sexual behaviour and in the possibilities for change to safer sex.

Sociologists, anthropologists and psychologists alike appeared ill prepared to meet these questions. It is astonishing how little we knew about actual sexual behaviour in Western societies, let alone in societies that have been less thoroughly researched (Caldwell et al. 1994; Holland et al. 1994). Caldwell et al. assume that sensitivity about the topic and misgivings about the respectability of studies in the field of sexual relations may have inhibited anthropologists from concentrating on sexual behaviour. If not only sexuality but also death is involved, the topic becomes even more sensitive. A further complication is the limited use for both personal and ethical reasons that can be made of participant observation, one of the most powerful social research methods. For insight into sexual practices we are dependent on what the actors tell us. Verification by observation is hardly possible, and counterchecking through interviews with partners also has its limitations: in many cases, particularly in non-marital relationships, the identity of the partner will not be revealed or cannot be traced (Caldwell et al. 1994; Pickering 1994; Pool 1997). Further methodological challenges concern the limited experience social scientists, including anthropologists, have with interviewing young adolescents, who are an important risk group for HIV infection, or with working in the sometimes risky surroundings where they may have to trace, for instance, commercial sex workers and their clients. Finally, the urgent quest for applicability of research findings challenges social science researchers.

AIDS induced social scientists to innovate in approaches, methods and fields of interest. Or rather: the need for AIDS-related social science research accelerated and enhanced developments that were already ongoing. One striking example is the interdiciplinarity of AIDS research. In all large research projects in Africa with which I am familiar, a variety of biomedical and social scientists – epidemiologists, clinical scientists, microbiologists, anthropologists, sociologists, health economists – cooperate.[5] The emphasis on participatory methods in the entire research process, including the application of results, is another example. Cooperation of researchers, health staff and community members in action research to support Primary Health Care has become increasingly common (CHRD 1990; Varkevisser 1996). AIDS research has been able to profit from these experiences, and to further develop lessons learned in the sensitive field of sexual research. The cross-cultural exploration of sexual relations and practices, the third innovative element, has perhaps been the greatest achievement of the social sciences in AIDS research. The accelerating AIDS pandemic also drew the attention of researchers and policy makers to the gender inequality in sexual relations, and highlighted the need to investigate the roots of this inequality in order to tailor AIDS interventions to the daily realities of women. This fourth new research development links up with ongoing gender research in other areas.

In the following sections I shall illucidate these innovations in social research. The illustrations come from sub-Saharan Africa, partly from the literature, partly from experience gained in the Tanzania-Netherlands Support Project for AIDS (TANESA). This is an interdisciplinary research and support project for AIDS interventions at district and regional level in Mwanza Region, Northwest Tanzania.[6]

Complementarity of epidemiological and social research

Epidemiological research reveals the magnitude and (geographical or social) distribution of problems. It also tests the strength of associations between problems and individual, potentially contributing factors. Sociologists and, in particular, anthropologists are more interested in *how* and *why* questions, in the development over time of epidemiologically established relationships and in the interrelatedness of different factors which influence a problem. One could say that epidemiological, quantitative data create the skeleton of a phenomenon, and that qualitative as well as quantitative data generated by social research provide the flesh for the bones.

The TANESA project started in 1989 with a prevalence survey in Mwanza region (pop. two million) among a geographically stratified sample of over 5000 people between 15 and 54 years old (Barongo et al. 1992). It was determined that HIV infection was highest (11.8%) in Mwanza town, the administrative centre of the region with some 250,000 inhabitants, moderate (7.3%) in smaller roadside settlements and lowest (2.5%) in rural areas. Moreover, HIV appeared to strike women at an earlier age than men: HIV prevalence was highest in women between 15 and 34 years, whereas in men most infections occurred between 25 and 44 years. These data supported plans for further research on the sexual behaviour of primary school pupils. Apart from the suggestions that differences in geographic mobility and a gender difference in the onset of sexual relations played a role in the manifestation of HIV in men and women,[7] the survey provided some further clues about risk factors for HIV infection. For men as well as women, marital status appeared significant: those single, widowed, separated or divorced had higher infection rates than those in stable relationships. The study also revealed an association between a past or present occurrence of a sexually transmitted disease (STD) and HIV, which led to further research into the nature of this link. For women, in particular, it showed a connection between being employed and HIV.

Social scientists analyzing these data usually come up with many additional questions which should help to explain the associations found by epidemiologists. What was the marital status of the women whose jobs put them at risk for HIV? What aspects in their working situation could explain their risk: skewed power relations with male employers, for example, which made it difficult to refuse sex with them, or the desire of women to exploit these unequal gender relations for money or improved career prospects? As a rule, additional research with a combination of various qualitative and quantitative techniques is necessary to answer such questions.

What sometimes surprises social scientists is the ease with which non-significant factors in epidemiological research end in the dustbin. The Mwanza survey revealed no association between religion and HIV infection, and the factor was dropped. However, one would at least have expected a difference between the sexual behaviour, and consequent HIV infection rates, of Christians whose religion condemns having multiple partners, compared with informants who are Muslim or adhere to traditional religions which are less restrictive in this respect. The fact that no such difference existed suggests that a century of preaching in favour of monogamy has had little effect.

Close cooperation between epidemiologists and social scientists is beneficial for both parties. Epidemiological research provides a basis for sub-samples to be used for further investigation of the many challenging questions that the data provoke. This saves medical anthropologists and sociologists time and helps to focus their study. They in turn may put the data of epidemiologists in a wider (cultural, socioeconomic, political) context. Such collaboration also helps to find direction for the application of research findings. With respect to evaluating changes in sexual behaviour, the cooperation between epidemiologists and anthropologists in the TANESA project proved essential in a study among factory workers.

In 1991, the epidemiologists started a cohort study among the 1750 workers of a factory in Mwanza town, in order to (1) follow changes over time in HIV incidence and (2) identify risk factors for HIV-1 seroconversion and for contracting other STDs. Furthermore, the study aimed at documenting possible changes in risk behaviour (reduction of partners and increase in condom use) after starting an intervention programme (Borgdorff et al 1994). Every four months, workers were asked to come to the factory clinic, which had been established by TANESA to support the study and render medical services to the labourers. During intake and follow-up visits, a standardized interview was carried out covering demographic and socio-economic variables, sexual behaviour and STDs/health. After the interview, respondents were physically examined, counselled if they wished, and serologically tested for HIV and syphilis. Treatment for STD and other reported diseases was free of charge. Condoms were also freely available. If the participants in the study wished, they could obtain the results of the HIV test and would be further counselled.[8] A fourth intervention included different health education activities: workshops for factory workers about AIDS, drama performance, and training and follow-up of peer health educators.

The social scientists of TANESA contributed to the content of the questionnaire – in particular to the sexual behaviour part of it – by using results of in-depth interviews with factory workers. Furthermore they shed light on commonly used terms which might be open to different interpretations, such as 'casual partner', 'regular partner', 'promiscuity' and 'prostitution', and assisted in providing depth and detail to the health education activities. As the second round of data from the cohort study came in, the epidemiologists also started asking some basic 'why' questions of the social scientists: what makes some labourers stick to one partner, whereas others continuously report that they have more than one; why do some labourers make use of the condoms provided, whereas others refuse to use them?

To answer these questions, the cohort study itself provided a useful basis. It was possible to select small samples of extremes: 10 workers who claimed to stick to one partner and 8 condom users, against 10 who reported having multiple partners and 8 who, despite risky behaviour, explicitly stated no use of condoms. As only 3% of the male and female labourers had recently used a condom (and only 15-18% had ever used one), it would have been extremely time- and labour-consuming to draw such a sample if the social scientists would have worked independently.

The cohort study had provided some clues as to who used condoms: the younger, better educated and higher income groups, and those who had recently suffered from STD. It also indicated when condoms were used: most frequently with casual partners (18% of casual contacts), much less with steady (non-marital) partners (2%), and hardly with spouses (0.2%) (Borgdorff et al. 1994). Subsequent informal interviews revealed many prejudices and dislikes of condoms which helped explain their low use. For example, the fear that they would burst and remain in the vagina, or that they were been infected with the HIV virus, or the dislike of reduced sensation. The association of condom use with loose sexual behaviour appeared a major factor responsible for their selective use. Asking a partner to use a condom could be perceived as either an accusation of unfaithfulness or a confession of infidelity, to which neither men nor women would aspire. As unfaithfulness on the woman's side is in the Mwanza region traditionally grounds for divorce, women will certainly hesitate to ask their partners to use condoms. For the sake of consolidating a new relationship, they may even ask their partners to stop using them:

> *Male, 28, single:*
> Since New Year, I have decided to have only one partner, a girl I met two weeks earlier. I have been using condoms with casual partners before, and also proposed my new partner to use condoms. But she was not happy with the idea and said that if I did not trust her, then we should part company (...) Since I had promised to marry the girl, I had to accept the situation, and we are not using condoms. (Nnko et al. 1993:11)

Cooperation between epidemiologists and social scientists became indispensable when the cohort study indicated that the factory workers were changing their sexual behaviour. Among 752 men who had visited the clinic five times over the years 1991-1994, the proportion which reported having had more than one sexual partner during the preceding month had gradually declined from 22.3 to 12.2%. The proportion of men reporting casual sex partners over the preceding month had almost halved: from 9.8 to 5.2% (Ng'weshemi et al. 1995). Were these changes real, or were they merely reflecting an increased awareness of desired sexual behaviour as a consequence of the health education activities in, and perhaps outside, the factory?

It was decided to use a number of tools to validate the findings of the cohort study: in-depth interviews (conducted by the social scientists) with a sub-sample of 45 factory workers, 20 of whom claimed to have changed their behaviour, against 25 reporting no change; cross-checks of the interview data of these 45 with the serological tests for HIV and with self-reported as well as clinically detected STDs (epidemiological data source). Where possible (in 10 cases), the wives of the selected factory workers were interviewed on the sexual behaviour of their husbands. Interviews were scrutinized for internal consistency as well as compared with each other.

Among the 20 factory workers who during the five successive rounds in the cohort study reported a reduction from many to few partners or had converted to monogamy, 16 were confirmed by all 'validation tools'. Only in four cases were there discrepancies in the different data sets.[9] These four were removed from the category 'changed behaviour', even though it cannot be excluded that HIV or STD infection may have been brought in by their partner instead of by their own risky behaviour. It appeared therefore that the change in number and type of partners reported in the cohort study was 'real'. Whether this change will in all cases be permanent is another question:

Male, 21, married with occasional casual partners:
I am still young. I may change my behaviour and involve myself in risks.
(Nnko et al. 1993:18)

A final example of how epidemiological and social science data can strengthen each other relates to the pre- or extramarital sexual behaviour of women. Only 13% of the 1750 factory workers in Mwanza among whom the cohort study took place were female. Compared with the men they were younger, more often single (never married) or divorced, and slightly better educated.[10] Given their relative youth and single status, one would have expected more risk behaviour among the women than among the men. Only a fraction of the female workers (4%), however, reported having had more than one partner in the past month, against 22% of the men. Whereas 71% of the men in the cohort study stated that they had ever had casual partners, this was mentioned by only 38% of the female workers. Focus group discussions with female factory workers indicated that women are hesitant to spoil their reputation and chances for marriage by openly admitting that they have had multiple, let alone casual partners.[11] In the cohort study in Mwanza, HIV infection rates confirmed the data of the FGDs: 17% of the female factory workers were infected with HIV, against 10% of the men, and thus it was clear that the women had underreported their risk behaviour. Subsequent qualitative research among school pupils revealed more details (see below).

In the Mwanza study, the epidemiologists and social scientists formed separate teams. In a similar study in Masaka district, Uganda, which started in 1988 and is still continuing, they formed one interdisciplinary team of researchers. That team carried out a population cohort study in 15 villages with demographic, socioeconomic, medical and serological components, on which many smaller studies have been based (Seeley et al. 1993). As a staunch supporter of health systems research in which such cooperation has proved to be very fruitful, I tend to opt for the one team approach. Most importantly, many researchers of different disciplines agree that a creative combination of different quantitative and qualitative techniques is required to study AIDS and sexual behaviour (Caldwell et al. 1994; Mulder 1996; Pickering 1994; Pool 1997; Power 1994).

Participative approaches in the study of adolescent sexual behaviour

Little was known about the sexual behaviour of young people when the AIDS epidemic began. In many societies adolescents are not supposed to engage in sexual activities, and certainly not to produce children before marriage. However, the increasing number of deaths and near deaths of young girls who were brought to hospital with complications of self-induced abortions in the 1980s alerted the medical services in the South to the fact that young girls and, likely, boys were sexually active, and that little was being done to guide them into safe sexual behaviour (Adjase 1997; Caldwell & Caldwell 1988; Coeytaux et al. 1993). Neither the maternal health services, which concentrated on married women, nor the schools had thus far paid much attention to the sexual education of young people. Traditional structures which used to prepare adolescents for adult life were eroding in many places. The alarming spread of AIDS and the high infection rates among, in particular, female teenagers further increased the urgency of action.

Western-oriented educators tend to mobilize teachers and parents as potential sexual educators for the youth. Yet it is doubtful whether these figures of authority are good sexual educators. In many societies, sexual matters are not easily discussed between parents and children (Caldwell et al. 1994). Older siblings, peers, sometimes grandparents or other relatives with whom children have a warm and joking relationship are much better suited to enlighten them on sexual health (Varkevisser 1973). When experimenting with various methods to reach the adolescents, not surprisingly the idea arose to use peers as sex educators.

Prior to starting any health education intervention, relevant messages have to be developed which are adapted to the knowledge, attitudes, emotions, behaviour and socio-economic possibilities of the target group. In the case of adolescents, these factors are all still developing. Neither peer educators nor their facilitators will therefore have sufficient background to develop adequate messages. The flexible use of different tools in combination may provide some insight into the knowledge, attitudes and behaviour of adolescents, but even then the research themes or questions are still determined by the researchers. The WHO Reproductive Health Programme recognised this as a problem and developed a *narrative research method* which allows the target group itself to determine the themes.

In its original form this method implies that youth leaders aged 18 to 25 are invited to participate in a workshop and develop their own story lines about how sexual relationships develop while role-playing. From the story lines, participants and facilitators generate questionnaires to acquire data. Workshop participants collect the data, which then are collectively analyzed and transformed into health education messages. These will be used by the participants to educate adolescents. The principle is that from the moment the research is being designed until the implementation of the end product, the participants themselves determine the content (WHO 1992, 1993).

Many variations of this method have been developed. In TANESA, the method was applied with involvement of three groups of about ten pupils from an upper primary school in Magu district: one group of boys, one of girls, and one mixed group of boys and girls. This set-up was chosen to provide an opportunity for gender-sensitive issues to be brought up. The facilitators were health educators/researchers with experience in facilitating role plays. The first days were spent on developing an atmosphere where sensitive issues could be openly discussed, on providing some knowledge on AIDS and reproductive health, and on explaining the exercise. Subsequently, the pupils developed story lines about typical encounters between boys and girls. Some themes were grouped together, after which the groups were asked to role-play the events. The role plays were video-taped and thoroughly analyzed for the meaning and motives of the actors. In this case, the sessions themselves formed the research situation, which was possible because the participants belonged to the target group from which they had been selected by their fellow pupils as future peer educators. In fact, this workshop formed the introduction to their training (Schapink et al. 1997).

When anthropologists in TANESA realized that observing acted sexual behaviour would be the closest possible substitute for observing real life situations (which would be a sheer impossibility), they invited male and female pupils from the higher classes of primary schools in Magu district (girls age 13 to 15, boys age 15 to 18) for separate role play workshops. The facilitators were near age-mates who had actively participated in an AIDS programme in a neighbouring secondary school. The pupils were requested to develop scripts based on significant episodes in adolescent relationships and then enact these. The performances were recorded on video and played back to the group for comment and discussion. These discussions, led by the *peer facilitators*, proved even more informative than the dialogues in the role plays. The discussions were tape-recorded and, like the role plays, transcribed and subjected to a rudimentary discourse analysis. A subsequent workshop of boys and girls did not bring new insights (Nnko & Pool 1995).

The results of role-play workshops were enlightening. Contrary to what parents and educational policy makers (who had been hesitant to include sexual education in the primary school curriculum as they feared it might encourage sexual activity) might expect or hope, a considerable proportion of 13-14-year-old pupils was already sexually active (Schapink et al. 1997). By the time they enter the higher classes of primary school, sexual education is therefore most timely. Though knowledge of HIV/AIDS and routes of infection was available, it did not serve as a deterrent for sexual contacts. Both girls and boys were much more afraid of unwanted pregnancies (see also Caldwell et al. 1994): girls, because they would have to leave school and face the anger of their parents; boys because of the possibility that their parents would have to pay compensation to the girls' parents, or that the girl's family would stress the obligation to marry the girl. Lust and curiosity would nevertheless often turn the scale in favour of sexual adventure, though girls would find many pretexts to postpone or dodge the encounter.

Even in these earliest sexual contacts there is gain involved for the girls: a little money, pens, writing books or cosmetics, acceptance of which would be regarded by the boy as willingness to cooperate. What is striking is the early age at which adolescents start exercising the adult skills of eloquence and negotiation in sexual contacts, the (often exaggerated) promises of presents, money, marriage from the side of the boy, and the calculated postponing on the side of the girl. Also surprising is the preference of girls for schoolboys initially, followed by slightly older men, who have more money, more experience and might become marriage partners. Preference was low for wealthy men the age of their fathers, who in AIDS education campaigns are often referred to as *sugar daddies*. In role plays, however, it was always girls from poorer families who became pregnant. This may indicate that their possibilities for negotiation and own partner choice are less, and the need for money is greater (Nnko & Pool 1995; Pool 1997; Schapink et al. 1997).

The strength of the *narrative research method* appears to be the participatory approach with emphasis on performance, which creates the possibility to gain insight into attitudes and behaviour of the target group that would otherwise remain largely concealed. Consequently, health education activities can be lifted from the level of stereotyped do's and don'ts to real *information, education and communication*, stressing the responsibility and possibilities for adolescents to protect themselves and their potential partners.

The socio-cultural context in which the method is applied does, of course, influence the modalities for application. Where premarital sexual relations are strictly condemned for girls and would bring shame to her family, the sheer discussion of the possibility would be likely to be considered an offense. Even in the Mwanza region, where traditionally premarital sex was silently condoned among the Sukuma (Varkevisser 1973), elaborate advocacy and sensitization of teachers, parents' committees and community leaders was required before the peer education programme could start in primary schools (Schapink et al. 1997). Preliminary research into the felt needs and possibilities for sexual education with all parties concerned, through key informant interviews and focus group discussions, seems an indispensable prelude to any sexual education programme and related social science research among young people.

Female sexual behaviour and management of sexual risks

Women deserve special attention with respect to HIV infection for several reasons. First, they appear more vulnerable than men to the virus.[12] Second, they are to a large, though widely varying, extent dependent on men for their social and economic well-being, due to the unequal distribution of resources and power between the sexes. Socioeconomic inequity between men and women is reflected in sexual relations. Even in Western societies some 30 years after the sexual revolution and despite equal opportunities for education and ever increasing participation of women in the labour market, this inequity is still noticeable in the sexual behaviour of young women and the risks they take (Holland et al. 1994). We can only try to understand such behaviour by analyzing its roots.

In any society rules exist to streamline sexual behaviour and fix rights and obligations between partners and their families. Since children resulting from sexual relationships guarantee the procreation of groups, this social concern is evident. Almost universally, marriages are contracts which are sealed by ceremonial exchange of gifts between families and partners, often sanctioned by religion. Though the content of the contract and the ceremony may have changed over time, they remain essential compasses for sexual behaviour.

In large parts of the world, marriage gives the husband the exclusive right to his wife's womb; in return he has to ensure protection, housing and economic support. In sub-Saharan Africa, where patrilineal descent is dominant, the family of the wife is compensated for the loss of a 'womb' with a bride-price. Sometimes the composition of the bride-price expresses the content of the contract, one (small) part entitling the husband to the exclusive sexual right, and another, much bigger part, entitling him and his lineage to the children born from the marriage.[13]

Though bride-price regulations are changing at present, the underlying notions may have been thoroughly internalized. These notions help explain the dependency of women on their husbands in decisions on sexual and reproductive behaviour, the difficulty to discuss (safe) sexual behaviour between spouses, and the reluctance of women, certainly when they are married, to report having possible sexual relations outside marriage to others.

If women have little or no power to influence the sexual behaviour of their partners on whom they are economically dependent, general messages such as 'reduce the number of partners' or 'use condoms' may have little relevance for them. What is worse: among women who have no other relations than with their partners, these messages may increase feelings of powerlessness instead of helping them to protect themselves.

Yet even in patrilineal societies, at least in sub-Saharan Africa, male rights to their wife's sexuality are not unlimited.[14] In the context of AIDS research into the loopholes in male power over female sexuality within marriages and regular relationships, and into possibilities for negotiating safer sex by women in these unions, is a priority. Thus far, the sexual behaviour of female sex workers and the possibilities for risk reduction have received much more attention from researchers and health educators than those of married women who are at risk through their partners. There may be several reasons for this preference. Sex workers were seen as a priority, because they had relatively high HIV infection rates and many sexual contacts through which they could further spread the virus. Though they may partly conceal their activities, sex workers have to 'go public' to attract customers. They can be identified and interviewed, provided sensitive and flexible techniques are used. Moreover, immediate action seems possible. Sex workers have most likely some flexibility in bargaining for safer sex, as men, if they use condoms, do so preferably in casual relations. Sex workers could be encouraged to exploit this opportunity. Marital relations, on the other hand, belong to the private domain. Both men and women may take the given power structures that underly sexual behaviour for granted. Discussing inequities would therefore have to involve women and men, in their role of husbands, fathers or, in matrilineal societies, mothers' brothers. A challenging, but not an easy task.

Research into prostitution in sub-Saharan Africa likewise has its challenges. The transition between prostitution and pre- or extramarital sex is vague. In fact, a wide range of sexual relations may exist between the extremes of prostitution – defined as full-time sex work, characterized by a fluctuating clientele, fixed prices, brothels and pimps who are entitled to part of the revenues – and having one lifetime partner. Prostitution so defined occurs, but as an exception (Caldwell et al. 1994). More common, though treated with discretion by girls, are premarital relationships. These in general start early in sub-Saharan Africa. Caldwell et al. (1994) cite many examples from the region; they stress the traditional reciprocity of the transaction: not being offered money or gifts would be an offence. Extramarital relations may occur as well, but are carefully hidden by women. The transactional component of such relationships can easily lead to confusion with prostitution.

In bigger towns, and along truck routes or other places with a concentration of mobile or single men, anonymous, commercialized sexual encounters have been increasing over the past decades. The majority of these activities are centered around local bars and beerhalls (Bassett et al. 1992; Meursing 1996; Mwizarubi et al. 1997). They are rarely full-time occupations. Wilson et al. (1990) made an inventory of sex work in and around bars and beerhalls in Bulawayo, Zimbabwe, and found that the women formed a cross-section of Bulawayo society, with widely varying education, incomes and occupations, though over 90% were either single or divorced. Mgalla & Pool (1996) identified the same characteristics among bar workers in the Mwanza Region. Even these casual sexual encounters, determined in the first place by the need for resources in the absence of other profitable alternatives, may turn into more permanent, more respectable and in an economic respect more reliable relationships.[15]

The complexity and sensitivity of the topic sexuality requires from researchers the keen nose of a tracker. Only bit by bit can they hope to unravel the truth. In such circumstances, surveys are, as Bleek has shown, unreliable tools.[16] More refined and varied armatory is required.

In a study in the Gambia among women who were engaged virtually full-time in sex work, Pickering (1994) and her research team used a combination of quantitative and qualitative tools. Questionnaires were given and daily records kept of the sexual behaviour of each of the 248 women in their sample. These were complemented by: interviews with 795 male clients, daily observations at the bars in which the women worked, in-depth interviews, visits to local markets (to observe whether lubricants and possibly harmful sexual stimulants were marketed, about the use of which the informants were hesitant to provide information), and visits to the homes of some of the sex workers. Moreover, a sample of 16 sex workers and a control group of 31 age-matched divorced or widowed women were asked to participate in daily monitoring of all their monetary transactions over a four-week period. As in the TANESA project, medical treatment was available from well supervised clinics which provided a basis of trust between interviewers and informants.

A careful comparison of data sources revealed, as could be expected, the unreliability and limited validity of one-time questionnaires. The estimates sex workers provided of the average daily number of clients appeared unreliable: they varied considerably over time and were twice as high as the numbers from the daily diaries and observations (which included nonworking days). Regarding the numbers of condoms used, the women gave a more rosy picture than their male clients, most likely because they assumed that their interviewers would lay high value on protection. The sex workers and their clients differed also in reports of the money that changed hands, the men mentioning much lower amounts.[17] A surprising finding was the relative wealth of at least some of the girls' parental homes, contradicting miserable stories of poverty and misfortune provided during the first interview. The height of their income compared very well to that of middle-rank civil servants and non-prostitute divorced and married women who supported themselves by informal sector activities as trading, cooking and selling food.[18]

The research findings confirm that cross-sectional surveys on (changes in) risk behaviour, whose results epidemiologists often use to make prognoses on the course of the AIDS epidemic, and health educators to evaluate their programs, may have limited value. Above all, the findings show that participative approaches are needed to develop the sort of messages and interventions from which women – and men – can profit.

The CONNAISSIDA action-research project in Zaire followed such an approach. In workshops including role plays followed by discussion, sex workers and, in a later stage, church women, followed by 'all male' and 'mixed sex' groups, searched for ways to ensure safer sexual behaviour adapted to the social context and lifestyles of the participants. Subsequent evaluations revealed how difficult it was for sex workers to maintain the high levels of condom use they acquired at the onset of the project: contradicting messages from church leaders and clients about the efficacy or desirability of condom use had demotivated them. It also appeared difficult to get marital partners to discuss sexual behaviour and adopt protective measures. Concern about the lives of their children had, however, notably decreased women's reluctance to discuss sexual matters with their partners (Schoepf et al. 1993).[19]

In an intervention project in Tanzania, coordinated by AMREF, which concentrates on long-distance truck drivers, bar/guesthouse workers, business men and workers at major construction sites, sex workers who had shown an interest in becoming peer educators were trained in interview techniques, and conducted in-depth interviews with colleagues selected through snowball sampling (Mwizarubi et al. 1997). As a result, thorough insight was obtained in sexual networking patterns and important transmission sites, as well as in risk behaviour such as anal intercourse which is not easily discussed with outsiders. This practice unfortunately appears to be on the increase, as many sexworkers and truck drivers consider it safer than vaginal sex (Mwizarubi et al. 1997; Pool 1997). The interviews by sex workers further revealed a rich variety of local expressions for sexual practices or clients' characteristics, which are one of the building stones for effective health education.

In Buluwayo, Zimbabwe, Wilson turned his research team into women pretending to be sex workers (Wilson et al. 1990). A team of volunteers, most of them nurses or students, who dressed themselves slightly frivolously in order to appear as unobtrusive as possible, visited all known beerhalls and bars at the end of the month. On employees' paydays, sex work is at its peak. The idea was to obtain a rather precise estimate of the magnitude of sex work, and thus a large number of interviewers were involved, who had to count all the girls or women acting at one point of time. Through informal discussion and by administering short individual questionnaires, a further attempt was made to identify who these women were (origin, marital status) and whether commercial sex work was a regular or an ad hoc activity for them. The study was related to an intervention programme, which included more in-depth research geared to strengthening the bargaining position of CSWs regarding condom use.

In the TANESA project an attempt was made to promote communication between men and women on safe sexual behaviour. Through a combination of drama, film or picture codes and discussions in female, male and mixed groups, daily problems which have their roots in gender inequality were analyzed. Another method used to influence gender relations is the *mapping exercise*. Two groups, one male, one female, work side by side, each developing a map of their village or urban community with major centres of social activity: markets, busstops, churches, schools, bars, health centres. Each group then defines places where they (would) feel at risk of contracting HIV. The groups also identify places where they can get information and services with respect to HIV and other STDs, and list problems and possibilities in avoiding risk behaviour. At the end, groups meet and discuss possible differences in conclusions (Balyagati & Schapink 1997).

The assumption underlying this approach is that the knowledge and awareness of inequities in gender relations should increase simultaneously in men and women, through mutual communication and, where necessary, confrontation. The role of social scientists in this process is that of reporter and moderator: asking, summarizing, contrasting, referring to relevant knowledge from other, similar discussions or from other sources. Information, education and communication (IEC) specialists usually carry the responsibility for turning the results into interventions like peer educator programmes and the development of information and training materials, though in close cooperation with the researchers and the target group. In TANESA intervention and research roles were partly separated and partly combined in the same person. Some social scientists switched from (predominantly) research to (predominantly) work on interventions.

Challenges we face

These new, participatory research approaches – and AIDS social science research in general – present us with many scientific and ethical challenges. The context of that research is, moreover, extremely difficult and stressful. Medical solutions are still very limited and costly, the economic situation, both at the national and personal level, is in many cases poor and deteriorating, and sociocultural conditions for behavioural change, which is usually a gradual process, are complex.

This research situation requires a number of adaptations from social scientists. First of all, they must be willing to cooperate with other scientists, both within their own broad field and beyond its disciplinary borders. This means working side by side with researchers of different backgrounds, understanding the research outcomes of other disciplines, the strengths and limitations of their research methods and, if appropriate, even participating in each others' activities. Evidently, such cooperation demands reciprocity.

There is a potential conflict between the different roles social scientists can take: that of researcher, translator of research data into messages or interventions, implementing IEC interventions, and evaluating them. It is impossible to carry out all these equally thoroughly: a choice in emphasis on research or implementation seems inevitable. Though ideally all should be involved in all activities, researchers focus better on preparation and evaluation of interventions. Translation of research results into action would be a shared responsibility with, for instance, IEC experts. Finding a balance between these different roles is a challenge, which can only be achieved by clear task descriptions and intensive cooperation.

Flexibility in the focus of research forms another challenge. As the pandemic progresses, new problems emerge. The research approaches described above mainly pertain to awareness raising and possible changes in sexual behaviour. With increasing HIV prevalence, the demands on relatives and the community and on health and social services for the care of patients increase. As the number of deaths rise, protection of widows and their children and the care of orphans become research issues. In sub-Saharan Africa, research in all these fields is ongoing, using traditional as well as more participatory methodologies. In other continents research in support of risk reduction is still in an early phase, and the problems to be faced may be different, e.g. child prostitution, stricter socioeconomic stratification, the larger size of the population at risk.

In all research, whether conducted by professional researchers or by lay (peer) researchers, the validity of the data collected should be a major concern. As a rule, researchers should work as a team, with a mix of insiders and outsiders inspiring each other into asking new questions and questioning the answers found. Regular discussion of the data obtained and adjustment of questions are obligatory, as building of knowledge is an iterative process.[20]

The need for careful selection and training of interviewers is evident. Seely et al. (1993) experimented with control interviews conducted from the same subjects with the same sets of questions or issues, in order to check whether there were differences in answers obtained by medical staff and social scientists, male and female interviewers of different ages. Some in formant-interviewer combinations were clearly unproductive: older women, for example, were reluctant to discuss sexual matters with young female researchers. Some differences were difficult to interpret: men mentioned more sexual partners vis-a-vis male interviewers than vis-a-vis females. Were they boasting or underreporting to make a good impression, or both? Seeley et al. advised keeping the social distance between informant and interviewer as low as possible, but some experimentation with reversed roles may be fruitful to learn about biases.

Care should be taken to include all relevant groups in the study: men and women, young and old, married and unmarried, traditional healers and health staff. It is interesting to note that many studies aiming at empowering women to exert more control over their lives exclude men (see Holland et al. 1994; Schoepf 1993).

The advantages of triangulation of different qualitative and quantitative methods through careful comparison of data acquired by different methods has already been mentioned. Feedback of major findings and conclusions to informants is another powerful tool to validate data which should form part of any study.

But the most important challenge is, I feel, of an ethical nature. Face to face with a fatal condition, one cannot stay impartial. Many of the studies mentioned are linked to the development or evaluation of interventions. Informants who express a need for information, counselling or treatment can be referred to services. Early recognition and treatment of STDs, especially in women where they are more hidden, reduces the risk of HIV infection (Grosskurth & Mwijarubi 1997). The TANESA project operates within the existing district governmental as well as non-governmental structures, and supports an integrated approach of research, health care, education and rural development activities. Working in a context of increasing gaps between rich and poor, of health services which lack money for voluntary HIV testing and provision of basic care to AIDS patients, the least one may ask of social researchers is to have a signalizing function.

Notes

1 In 1992 this was a reason to shift the location of the Global Conference on AIDS from the USA to the Netherlands, where, like in other member states of the EU, such an obligation did not exist.

2 Quinn (1996) estimates that worldwide over 75% of all HIV infections occur through unprotected sex. The fact that more women than men are at present HIV positive in sub-Saharan Africa indicates the importance of heterosexual transmission. The mother to child transmission rate in Africa is roughly 25%, with variations from 20-45% (Urassa et al. 1997).

3 Sometimes local newspapers reflected dubious Western sources. The journal *New African* in its September 1996 issue supported Neville Hodgekinson's book *AIDS, the failure of contemporary science; how a virus that never was deceived the world*. The *New African* also raised the question whether African attempts to find a cure for AIDS were being frustrated to create a market for Western drug companies.

4 UNAIDS/WHO (1997) estimates that this number has already been reached by the end of 1997.

5 For example: the World Bank sponsored project *The economic impact of fatal adult illness due to AIDS and other causes in sub-Saharan Africa* in Kagera region, Tanzania; the *Tanzania-Netherlands project to support AIDS control in Mwanza region, Tanzania*, the Medical Research Council Programme on AIDS in Uganda (Masaka District), the Medical Research Council Programme on AIDS in the Gambia, all have employed interdisciplinary research teams. A study on child sexual abuse in Matabeleland, Zimbabwe, spontaneously emerged as a cooperative effort of concerned psychologists, public health physicians, clinicians, medical sociologists, nurses and lawyers (Meursing et al. 1995).

6 TANESA is implemented by the Government of Tanzania, financed by the Netherlands Ministry of Foreign Affairs and technically supported by the Royal Tropical Institute, Amsterdam. In an earlier phase the acronym TANERA was used.

7 See Barongo et al. (1994) on the relationship between mobility of men and HIV infection. With respect to onset of sexual activity, Borgdorff et al. (1994) found in a cohort study among factory workers that, contrary to expectations, men reported having sexual contacts at an earlier age than women. This finding was contradicted by further qualitative research.

8 By 1994, only 10% of the participants had, however, done so, and among these the HIV-positive labourers were underrepresented. Of the 926 male factory workers who enrolled in the first round, 91 (10%) were HIV positive, against 37 (17%) of the 217 females (170 labourers and 37 spouses of male labourers). Of the 128 HIV positives, only 6 (5%) came for the results, whereas on the whole, 148 (13%) of the 1143 investigated persons came (Barongo et al. 1994).

9 In one case, the in-depth interview revealed extramarital partners who had not appeared in the survey. In the three remaining cases, one respondent became sero-positive despite his reported monogamous behaviour, another developed an STD, and the wife of the third said her husband had had extra-marital partners during the period he claimed not to have had them (Pool et al. 1996).

10 Of the 170 women enrolled in the cohort study, one-third were between 15 and 24 years old against only 16% of the 926 men; 18% had completed secondary education, compared with 13% of the men, and only 42% were married, against 77% of the men (unpublished data cohort study).

11 Such underreporting is also confirmed by other authors for sub-Saharan Africa, e.g. Caldwell et al. (1994).

12 Sherr (1996:22) concludes that the risk of transmission after a single unprotected act of intercourse between an HIV-positive woman and a man is 2-20 times less likely than is transmission from an HIV-positive man to a woman. See also Mgalla et al. 1997.

13 Among the Sukuma in Tanzania, for example, one bull for the 'nuptial hut' secured the husband the exclusive sexual possession of his wife. One cow and a bull, the 'cows of departure', conferred on a man the prerogative to take his wife with him to his homestead where she would work and cook for him and his relatives. The remaining cattle (1-15, depending on the age and status of the woman) allowed the husband and his relatives to attribute the offspring born from the marriage to their descent group (Varkevisser 1973).

14 Caldwell et al (1994) stress that in Western sub-Saharan Africa, pre- and post partem taboos on sexual intercourse still reduce the period in which a husband has the right to approach his wife sexually in her reproductive phase considerably, whereas in Eastern Africa this custom has eroded much more quickly. They hypothesize that this difference may be associated with the lower prevalence of STDs, infertility and HIV among Western African women compared with Central and Eastern Africa.

15 Wilson et al. (1990) mention that over half of the clients of bar-based respondents were repeat clients. They do not state whether this influenced the mode of payment, but mention that sometimes no money would be paid. Mgalla & Pool (1996) observed that in a regular relationship the financial support became more general, according to the financial needs of the women, instead of payment in direct exchange for sex. These regular partners were mostly married men, which minimized the chances for a real marriage.

16 Bleek (1987) found that girls and young women in a Ghanean village who were interviewed by local nurses with a standard questionnaire about their sexual relations and experiences with (illegal) abortion provided answers which were quite deviant from the far more detailed and complicated pictures he had managed to construct during six months of participant observation in the same village.

17 Pickering (1994) assumes that the CSWs were unwilling to admit that they had accepted prices below the standard set between themselves, but the men – when questioned in-depth about the discrepancies – gave a different explanation: fear of clients to admit that they had squandered such a high proportion of their (family) income on prostitutes.

18 This finding and the also reported limited inclination among CSWs to invest in the informal sector indicate that income-generating activities or credit facilities for women may be more effective to prevent or limit prostitution, than to bring women who have commercial sex as a main source of income back to the path of honour. Saving facilities and advice on investment might be at least as appropriate for commercial sex workers.

19 Likewise, the MRC Programme on AIDS in Uganda critically experimented with different, increasingly intense levels of community participation in the studies conducted. Here the results were translated into individual and community counselling activities, in close cooperation with The AIDS Support Organisation (TASO), one of the first self-help groups in Uganda (Seeley et al. 1992).

20 Preferably, interviews should be taped, or data should be saved by taped discussions of team members of what they have seen and heard immediately after an interview.

Literature

Adjase, E.T.
 1997 *Hu m'ani so ma me ti. Teenage sexuality, unwanted pregnancy and the consequences of unsafe abortion in Sunyani District, Ghana.* MPH Thesis. Amsterdam: Royal Tropical Institute.

Balyagati, D. & D. Schapink
 1997 'Addressing gender and gender-related issues.' In: J. Ng'Weshemi, T. Boerma, J. Bennett & D. Schapink (eds), *HIV prevention and AIDS care in Africa. A district level approach.* Amsterdam: KIT Press, pp. 150-162.

Barnett, T. & P. Blaikie
 1992 *AIDS in Africa: Its present and future impact. London: Belhaven.*

Barongo, L.R., M.W. Borgdorff, F.F. Mosha, A. Nicoll, H. Grosskurth, K.P. Senkoro et al.
 1994 'The epidemiology of HIV-I infection in urban areas, roadside settlements and rural villages in Mwanza Region, Tanzania.' In:
   M. Borgdorff, *Epidemiology of HIV-I infection in Mwanza region, Tanzania.* Amsterdam: KIT Press. pp. 40-52.

Borgdorff, M.W., L.R. Barongo, J.N. Newell, K.P. Senkoro, W. Devillé,
J.P. Velema & R.M. Gabone
1994   'Sexual partner change and condom use among urban factory workers in
northwest Tanzania.' In: M.W. Borgdorff, *Epidemiology of HIV-1 infection in Mwanza region, Tanzania.* Amsterdam: KIT Press, pp. 99-111.

Bleek, W.
1987   'Lying informants: A fieldwork experience from Ghana.' *Population &
Development Review* 13(2): 314-22.

Boulton, M. (ed.)
1994   *Challenge and innovation: Methodological advances in social research on
HIV/AIDS.* London: Taylor & Francis.

Caldwell, J.C. & P. Caldwell
1988   *Marital status and abortion in sub-Saharan Africa.* Paper for the IUSSP
Seminar on Nuptiality in sub-Saharan Africa, Paris.

Caldwell, J.C., I.O. Orubuloye & P. Caldwell
1992   'Underreaction to AIDS in sub-Saharan Africa.' *Social Science & Medicine*
34(11): 1169-1182.

Caldwell, J.C., I.O. Orubuloye & P. Caldwell
1994   'Methodological advances in studying the social context of AIDS in West
Africa.' In: I.O. Orubuloye, J.C. Caldwell, P. Caldwell & G. Santow,
*Sexual networking and AIDS in sub-Saharan Africa: Behavioural research
and the social context.* Canberra: Health Transition Centre, pp. 1-12.

Caldwell, J.C., P. Caldwell & P. Quiggin
1994   'The social context of AIDS in sub-Saharan Africa.' In: I.O. Orubuloye,
J.C. Caldwell, P. Caldwell & G. Santow, *Sexual networking and AIDS in
sub-Saharan Africa: Behavioural research and the social context.* Canberra:
Health Transition Centre. pp. 129-62.

Commission on Health Research for Development (CHRD)
1990   *Health research: Essential link to equity in development.* Oxford: OUP.

Coeytaux, F.M., A.H. Leonard & C.M. Bloomer
1993   'Abortion.' In: M. Koblinsky, J. Timyan & J. Gay, *The health of women:
A global perspective.* Boulder: Westview Press, pp. 133-46.

Farmer, P.
1992   *AIDS and accusation. Haiti and the geography of blame.* Berkeley: University of California Press.

Farmer, P.
1996   'Women, Poverty and AIDS.' In: P. Farmer, M. Connors & J. Simmons
(eds), *Women, poverty and AIDS: Sex, drugs and structural violence.*
Monroe: Common Courage Press, pp. 1-33.

Holland, J., C. Ramazanoglu, S. Scott, S. Sharpe & R. Thomson
1994 'Methodological Issues in researching young women's sexuality.' In: M. Boulton (ed.), *Challenge and innovation: Methodological advances in social research on HIV/AIDS.* London: Taylor & Francis, pp. 219-40.

Madraa, E. & Ruranga-Rubaramira
1996 *HIV prevention works: The Uganda case study. Paper for the* ixth International Conference on AIDS in Vancouver, July 1996.

Mann, J.M., & D.J.M. Tarantola (eds)
1996 AIDS *in the world II: Global dimensions, social roots, and responses. New York:* OUP.

Meursing, K., T. Vos, O. Coutinho, M. Moyo, S. Mpofu, V. Mundy, S. Dube, T. Mahlangu & F. Sibindi
1995 'Child sexual abuse in Matabeleland, Zimbabwe.' *Social Science & Medicine* 41(12): 1693-1704.

Meursing, K.
1997 *A world of silence: Living with* AIDS *in Matabeleland, Zimbabwe.* Amsterdam: KIT Press.

Mgalla, Z., L. Wambura & M. de Bruyn
1997 'Gender and HIV/AIDS.' In: J. Ng'weshemi, T. Boerma, J. Bennett & D. Schapink (eds), *HIV prevention and AIDS care in Africa. A district level approach.* Amsterdam: KIT Press, pp. 85-100.

Mulder, D., A. Nunn, A. Kamali & J. Kengeya-Kayondo
1995 'Decreasing HIV-1 seroprevalence in young adults in a rural Ugandan cohort.' *British Medical Journal* 311: 833-836.

Mulder, D.W.
1996 *The epidemiology of HIV-1 in a rural Ugandan population.* PhD Thesis. Rotterdam: Erasmus University.

Ng'weshemi, J., T. Boerma, L. Barongo, K. Senkoro, R. Isingo & M. Borgdorff
1995 *Changes in male sexual behaviour in response to the* AIDS *epidemic: Quantitative evidence from a cohort study in urban Tanzania.* TANESA Working Paper no. 6. Mwanza:TANESA.

Ng'weshemi, J., T. Boerma, J. Bennett & D. Schapink (eds)
1997 *HIV prevention and* AIDS *care in Africa: A district level approach.* Amsterdam: KIT Press.

Nnko, S., J. Mwanga, C. Varkevisser, M. Borgdorff, B. Chiduo, M. Dautzenberg & G. Lwihula
1993 *Risk perception and behavioural change in relation to* AIDS. TANERA, Unpublished report.

Nnko S., & R. Pool
1995 *School pupils and the discourse of sex in Magu District, Tanzania.* TANESA Working Paper no. 3. Mwanza: TANESA.

Orubuloye, I.O., J.C. Caldwell, P. Caldwell & G. Santow
  1994   *Sexual Networking and AIDS in sub-Saharan Africa: Behavioural research and the social context.* Canberra: Health Transition Centre.
Pickering, H.
  1994   'Social science methods used in a study of prostitutes in the Gambia.' In: M. Boulton (ed.), *Challenge and innovation: Methodological advances in social research on HIV/AIDS.* London: Taylor & Francis, pp. 149-58.
Pool, R., M. Maswe, T. Boerma & S. Nnko
  1996   *The price of promiscuity: Why urban males in Mwanza are changing their sexual behaviour.* TANESA Working Paper no. 8. Mwanza: TANESA.
Pool, R.
  1997   'Anthropological research on AIDS.' In: J. Ng'weshemi, T. Boerma, J. Bennett & D. Schapink (eds), *HIV prevention and AIDS care in Africa. A district level approach.* Amsterdam: KIT Press. pp. 69-85.
Power, R.
  1994   'Some methodological and practical implications of employing drug users as indigenous fieldworkers.' In: M. Boulton (ed.), *Challenge and innovation: Methodological advances in social research on HIV/AIDS.* London: Taylor & Francis, pp. 97-109.
Quinn, T.C.
  1996   'Global burden of the HIV pandemic.' Lancet 348: 99-106.
Schapink D., J. Hema & B. Mujaya
  1997   'Youth and HIV/ AIDS programmes.' In: J. Ng'weshemi, T. Boerma, J. Bennett & D. Schapink (eds), *HIV prevention and AIDS care in Africa. A district level approach.* Amsterdam: KIT Press. pp. 163-84.
Schoepf, B.G., W. Engunda, R. wa Nkera, P. Ntsomo & C. Schoepf
  1993   'Empowerment through risk reduction workshops.' In: M. Berer & S. Ray (eds), *Women and HIV/AIDS. An international resourcebook.* London: Harper Collins Publishers. pp. 219-24.
Seely, J.A., J.F. Kengeya-Kayondo & D.W. Mulder
  1992   'Community-based HIV/ AIDS research – whither community participation? Unsolved problems in a research programme in rural Uganda.' *Social Science & Medicine* 34(10): 1089-1095.
Seely, J., P. Huygens, E. Kajura, U. Wagner & D. Mulder
  1993   *Issues in interviewing individuals about sexual behaviour: Implications for interviews.* Paper presented at the London School of Hygiene and Tropical Medicine, 19th October 1993.
The Sunday Times, 3 October 1993: The plague that never was.
Todd, J. & L. Barongo
  1997   'Epidemiological methods.' In: J. Ng'weshemi, T. Boerma, J. Bennett & D. Schapink (eds), *HIV prevention and AIDS care in Africa. A district level approach.* Amsterdam: KIT Press. pp. 51-68.

UNAID/WHO
1997   *Report on the global AIDS epidemic.* Geneva: UNAIDS/WHO.

Urassa, M., G. Walraven & T. Boerma
1997   'Consequences of the AIDS epidemic for children.' In: J. Ng'weshemi,
       T. Boerma, J. Bennett & D. Schapink (eds), *HIV prevention and AIDS care
       in Afrika. A district level approach.* Amsterdam: KIT Press, pp. 337-49.

Varkevisser, C.M.
1973   *Socialization in a changing society: Sukuma childhood in rural and urban
       Mwanza, Tanzania.* Den Haag: Centre for the Study of Education in
       Changing Societies.
1996   *Health Systems Research: De knikkers en het spel.* Amsterdam: Royal
       Tropical Institute.

Wilson, D., B. Shibanda, L. Mboyi, S. Msimanga & G. Dube
1990   'A pilot study for an HIV intervention programme among commercial sex
       workers in Bulawayo, Zimbabwe.' *Social Science & Medicine* 31(5):
       609-618.

World Health Organization
1992   *A study of the sexual experience of young people in eleven African coun-
       tries.* Adolescent Health Programme. Geneva: WHO.
1993   *The narrative research method. Studying behaviour patterns of young
       people by young people. A guide to its use.* Adolescent Health Programme.
       Geneva: WHO.

CHAPTER V

Medical Interventions for Safe Motherhood: Options for a Broader Approach

J.A. Kusin

Ten years after the Safe Motherhood Initiative (SMI) was launched, the deaths of 600,000 women per year from pregnancy-related complications continue to be a reality (WHO/UNICEF 1996). Ninety-nine percent of those deaths take place in the developing world, 89% in Africa and South Asia alone (Koblinsky et al. 1995). Recently, maternal mortality rates (MMR) have been grouped within a country's Human Development Index (HDI), composed of a weighted ratio of life expectancy at birth, educational attainment and income, that is the real GDP by dollar parity (UNDP 1996). The significant relation between HDI and MMR in developing countries clearly illustrates the link between socio-economic development and MMR: the range for low, medium and high HDI countries was 548, 161 and 67 per 100,000 live births, respectively. The corresponding figure for the industrial countries is 10 per 100,000 live births. However, at the same level of HDI, a wide range of maternal mortality was recorded, suggesting that what matters is the allocation of resources to appropriate programmes. Why has reproduction, the most natural and physiological feature of human life, become a nightmare of potential death? What are the medical possibilities to achieve safe motherhood, which implies a reduction of maternal mortality and morbidity, and an enhancement of the survival and health of newborn infants. Mortality is preceded by ill health. This paper will focus on non-infectious morbidity of women of reproductive age, i.e. nutritional deprivation and its consequences.

Maternal mortality and undernutrition

Maternal deaths can be classified as *indirect* (pre-existing such as malaria, anaemia, made worse by pregnancy) and *direct* obstetric deaths due to complications of pregnancy, delivery or the postpartum period. The vast majority of maternal deaths (75%) fall in the latter category of which 20-35% can be attributed to haemorrhage, 20-45% to induced abortion/teenage pregnancy, 15-25% to hypertension/eclampsia, 5-15% to infection/sepsis, and 5-15% to obstructed labour (Maine 1991; Tinker & Koblinsky 1993).

It is known that the nutritional status of a woman (current and past) is an important determinant of the ease with which she will carry the fetus to term, and of the likelihood that she and the infant will survive and emerge from the delivery in good health with the capacity to breast feed successfully (Kusin & Jansen 1986; Kusin & Kardjati 1994; Norton 1994). Poor maternal nutritional health contributes to at least four of the five major causes of maternal mortality. Blood loss during delivery has much more serious consequences in anaemic women and the risk of dying is far greater. Maternal infection may be exacerbated by even mild iron and vitamin A deficiencies which lead to reduced immuno-competence (Stolzfus 1994).[1] Sepsis is also attributable to prolonged labour due to chronic energy deficiency (a major cause of low birth weight, i.e. 24 million infants in 1993). Small stature as a result of childhood malnutrition is a recognized risk for obstructed labour and contributes to the widespread preference for small newborns. It is therefore understandable that in many cultures women tend to reduce food intake during pregnancy (Hutter 1994; Kusin et al. 1984; Kusin & Kardjati 1994). Among those who survive prolonged or obstructed labour, many are permanently disabled because of the fistula developed. WHO estimates that about 80,000 women are affected each year and about 500,000 to 1 million women were living with the problem in 1995. The nutritional link with eclampsia is still tentative. Almost all dietary surveys report extremely low calcium intakes in poor communities which cannot afford milk and milk products. There is compelling evidence that high calcium intake reduces the likelihood of developing eclampsia (Bucher et al. 1996a, 1996b).

Due to a lack of good epidemiological data on nutritional status among adults the extent of nutritional deficiencies among women in the developing world is unknown. Quite conservative estimates suggest that among the 1,130 million women aged 15-60 years in the developing countries in 1985, over 500 million were anaemic, about the same number were stunted, almost 100 million have frank goitres, and some 200 million were vitamin A deficient. It is not likely that this situation has improved in the last decade (Leslie 1994; WHO 1996a).

Reproduction and maternal depletion

It is obvious that infant and maternal survival, health and well-being are best in communities which are well-fed. In developing countries 20-60% of women of reproductive age are marginally nourished to start with. Most food consumption surveys in developing countries show that women have an energy intake of 1500-1700 kcal/day (70% of requirement) and a protein intake of about 42 g per day (85% of requirement): too much to die, too little to live a healthy and active life. Undernutrition among women of reproductive age is caused by a discrimination in terms of food allocation, the heavy burden of productive activities requiring physical labour and the extra nutritional demands of reproduction. These determinants of women's nutritional status are in turn influenced by a range of cultural, social and economic factors (McGuire & Popkin 1989).

UNFPA's risk profile *too young, too many, too close and too old* summarizes the well-recognized nutritional risk due to reproduction (WHO 1996b). The stark difference between the cost of reproduction for women in industrial countries (and their affluent counterparts in the Third World) and that of poor women in developing countries is illustrated in Table 1. The calculation is based on median figures for menarche (age at first menstruation) and menopause (age when women stop menstruating).

Contrary to the myth that women in developing countries are more fertile, the fecundity (ability to reproduce) of poor women is much lower than that of women raised and living in a healthy environment, well-nourished from early childhood. As menarche is earlier in well-nourished girls and menopause later in well-nourished women, the fertile period is about 1,5 times longer than among undernourished women. The number of pregnancies and the decision to breast feed, particularly how long to breast feed, also differ clearly. Women in industrial countries deliver only 2 children and usually breast-feed for a period of 4 months or less. They hence spend about 5% of their fertile period on reproduction. In contrast, women in poor communities have more children, in this calculation 6 children and prolonged breast feeding is still the rule, particularly in rural areas. As a result, they are pregnant and/or lactating for 59% of their fertile period. In traditional communities with low contraceptive use women tend to stop breast feeding when they notice that they are pregnant from fetal movements in their womb. As these occur at about 4 months of pregnancy, an appreciable overlap between pregnancy and lactation occurs (Merchant et al. 1990), increasing the nutritional stress on mothers. The sequential burden of reproduction on the women's health and nutritional status is known as the *maternal depletion syndrome*.

Table 1 Maternal depletion: child bearing and nurturing as percent of reproductive period

Variables	Developing countries*	Industrial countries**
Menarche, age	14	11
Menopause, age	42	53
Fertile period, years	28	42
Number of children	6	2
months pregnant	6 × 9 = 54	2 × 9 = 18
months lactating	6 × 24 = 144	2 × 4 = 8
Months reproducing		
- total	198 m = 16.5 years	26 m = 2+ years
- as percent of fertile period	59%	5%

* poor sections of the population
** excluding deprived population groups

Consequences of chronic energy deficiency

Safe motherhood implies physiological reproduction, more than maternal mortality. It entails satisfactory infant outcomes (birth weight, the quantity and quality of breast milk) as well as maternal outcomes (survival, health and no depletion).

Of all deficiencies, the most important is chronic energy deficiency (CED), defined by a body mass index (BMI=kg/m^2) of less than 18.5 (James et al. 1988). It serves as an indicator of poverty which determines the amount and type of foods consumed. The consequences of the maternal depletion syndrome is illustrated by the biological processes occurring during CED.

Adequate childbearing and breast feeding can occur in association with a wide range in dietary intake. However, it has been demonstrated that the size of the baby born to undernourished mothers can be 200-300 g less than those delivered by well-nourished mothers (Andersson & Bergstrom 1997; Pitkin 1990), and growth faltering may start as early as the third month of intrauterine life (Kolsteren 1996). The range in the incidence of low birth weight (< 2500 g) is 11-25% in developing countries, 40-60% in the Indian subcontinent and less than 6% in industrial countries and affluent communities in the Third World (UNICEF 1997). The quantity of breast milk produced appears to be better protected (Prentice et al. 1994), but the composition (notably fat, vitamin, mineral content) may be impaired (Kusin & Kardjati 1994).

These average figures conceal the repercussions of CED as infant and maternal outcomes of reproduction have not been analyzed by the degree of maternal energy depletion. Our studies of pregnant and lactating women in East Java and Madura, Indonesia, over a period of over 10 years suggest that BMI as an indicator of CED in women is predictive for impairment of reproductive function. The longitudinal study started with baseline surveys in 1976-77 and 1980, followed by an experimental trial of food supplementation during the last trimester of pregnancy in 1981-85 and a follow-up of mother-infant pairs in 1986-90.[2] In summary, the framework of the study was a surveillance of all mothers with children, age 0-60 months, and newly married couples through 4-weekly home visits. During these visits, body measurements of mothers (irrespective of their reproductive status) were taken, and they were asked whether they menstruated or not, to detect a pregnancy. Birth weight was measured within 24 h after delivery. After birth, mother-child pairs were monitored (weight, height of everyone, dietary intake, breast milk production, morbidity, activity patterns in subsamples) until the child was 3 years old.

These studies showed that in East Java 23% of women of reproductive age were chronically energy deficient. It was much more common on the poorer island Madura where the longitudinal study was conducted, namely 37%. There was a downward gradient in incidence of low birth weight in women with a pre-pregnant BMI of less than 16, 16-17, 17-18.5 and over 18.5 (not CED), namely 22%, 10%, 8% and 5% (similar to well-nourished populations). In addition, the weight gain of infants in the first 6 months (indicator of breast milk production) was 3280 g and 3520 g for those born to CED and non-CED mothers, respectively. However, there was an inverse relation between maternal weight gain and birth weight or infant growth in the first 6 months across BMI categories. Mothers with a pre-pregnant BMI < 17 gained about 2.5 kg in pregnancy, while those with a BMI ≥18.5 did not gain any weight or lost weight! The same observation was made during lactation. The most depleted mothers after delivery (BMI< 16) gained about 1.3 kg in the first 6 months, the non-CED mothers lost about 0.7 kg! Thus, the more energy deficient the mother, the more available energy (food intake) was used to recuperate (replenish fat stores) at the expense of fetal growth and lactation! How much of available energy was channelled to the mother and the fetus, or the mother and breast milk, depended on the degree of CED of the mother (Kusin et al. 1994). It is, therefore, obvious that the impact of an intervention such as supplementary feeding during pregnancy and/or lactation depends on the degree of maternal depletion and the targeted outcome. Favourable infant outcomes can only be achieved after mothers have replenished their body fat status (BMI>18.5). Consequently, it is unrealistic to expect an improvement in infant outcomes of pregnancy unless maternal outcomes are secured.

Increasingly, evidence suggests that even the long-term health of adults is influenced by their weight at birth and early infancy, which as shown above is related to safe motherhood. It appears that a stimulus or insult in the sensitive period of fetal life and infancy programmes a long-term change in structure or function of an organ (Barker 1992). Studies in the UK and India show that small size at birth is associated with ischaemic heart disease (IHD), hypertension, stroke, diabetes and chronic bronchitis while in the UK the shortest people have the highest rates of deaths from IHD, stroke and chronic bronchitis (Martyn et al. 1996; Stein et al. 1996). Thus, maternal undernutrition has profound consequences on maternal mortality, infant survival and development, and adult non-infectious morbidity. Maternal undernutrition maintains the inter-generation cycle of poor nutrition and health.

Is reproduction the sole culprit of women's poor nutrition?

Undoubtedly, reproduction is an important nutritional stress for women, but it is a false assumption that family planning would solve the nutritional problems in pregnancy and lactation. Such will only be the case if women start their first pregnancy with an adequate nutritional status. The period immediately preceding reproduction is adolescence. It is the period of passing from childhood to adulthood which is defined as early adolescence from 10-14 years and late adolescence from 15-19 years (WHO 1990). It is estimated that in 1992 about 750 million of the world's population are in the age group 10-19 years and more than 80% of the world's youth live in developing countries. Adolescence is characterised by a second growth spurt and thus higher energy and nutrient requirements. An additional nutritional demand is created if pregnancy and lactation are superimposed on a still growing adolescent. There is a great lack of health and nutritional information of adolescents worldwide and particularly in developing countries. The multi-country study sponsored by the International Center for Research on Women in Washington DC was a first effort to systematically document adolescent nutritional status (Kurz & Johnson-Welch 1994). Stunting (less than 5th percentile NCHS/WHO height-for-age) was prevalent in 9 of 11 studies, ranging from 27-65%. Only one study (India) showed worse female stunting. Thinness (less than 5th percentile NCHS/WHO BMI-for-age) was equally high in 3 of 11 studies, ranging from 23-53%, with a gender bias in favour of girls. Anaemia was the greatest nutritional problem in 4 of the 6 studies in which it was assessed, range 32-55%.

The surveys conducted in East Java by the School of Medicine, Airlangga University, Surabaya, and our team mentioned earlier covered mothers and their children in the age group 0-15 years. Figures 1-3 show that mean weight, height and BMI of the Indonesian children in Madura and East Java are much lower than that of the NCHS/WHO reference (Dibley et al. 1987).

Figure 1 Weight by age

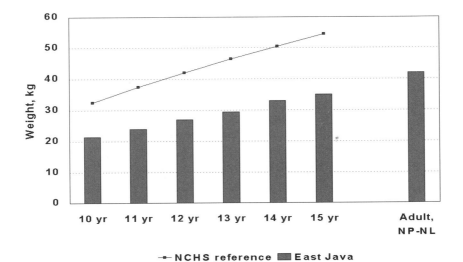

Figure 2 Height by age

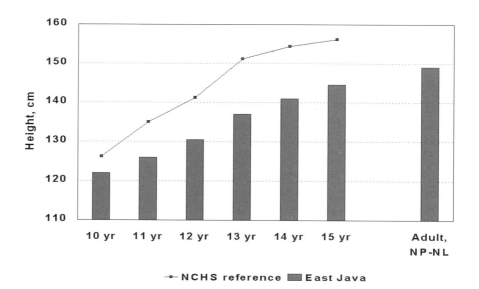

Figure 3 BMI by age

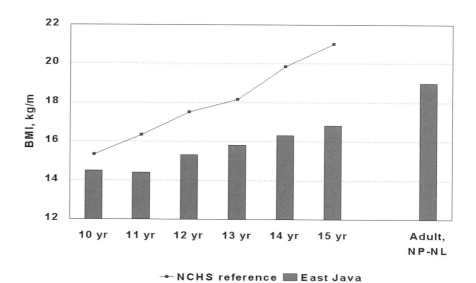

Even if the difference in mean menarchal age is taken into consideration (USA children around 12 years and Indonesian children around 15 years), the data illustrate that Indonesian children are not only stunted (low height-for-age) but also very lean. Comparison with their mothers indicates that low adult height, weight and BMI are a reflection of CED in early childhood and adolescence.

Data from the longitudinal study of nutrition during pregnancy in Madura in the years 1981-1990 (Kusin & Kardjati 1994) showed that CED was quite common among primiparae. Unexpectedly, BMI was not worse in the higher parity groups nor related to birth interval (Table 2). Such a pattern suggests that a number of primiparae are adolescents, which is quite probable. At the time of our study, modern contraception was not common and parity was closely related to age. The prevalence of *hypovitaminosis A* (serum levels less than 20 microgram/100 ml) and anaemia were in the same range for children 10-15 years of age and their mothers (Table 3). The significant observations are (i) the regional poverty-related differences, Madura being worse off in all aspects than the rest of East Java, and (ii) the magnitude of micronutrient deficiency in the age group 10-15 years. Already about 45% had low levels of vitamin A levels and 23-40% suffered from anaemia. It is obvious that the nutritional inadequacy starts before reproduction and is at least as important, probable even more important, than the nutritional stress due to reproduction.

Table 2 Pre-pregnant BMI by parity and birth interval, Madura 1981-90

Variables	Parity		
	1	2-5	≥ 6
number % CED*	93	776	216
	47	39	30
	Birth interval, months**		
	< 18 m	18-27 m	≥ 28 m
number % CED	77	204	467
	32	42	34

* CED = chronic energy deficiency, Body Mass Index < 18.5
** Birth interval: number of months between current and preceding birth

The surveys in East Java were conducted two decades ago. It is, however, very probable that the nutritional status of adolescents has not changed much between the late 1970s and the 1990s, as is the case for preschool children and women of reproductive age (Kardjati 1992; Kodiat 1994). One may conclude that the nutritional stress during reproduction is superimposed on the poor nutritional status during adolescence and early childhood.

Table 3 Prevalence of hypovitaminosis A and anaemia by age, physiological state and area (surveys 1976-1977)

Age or physiological state	Serum vit A < 20 ug%		Anaemia	
	East Java	Madura	East Java	Madura
Children				
10-12 yr	49%	45%	30%	40%
13-15 yr	41%	47%	22%	23%
Women				
* NP-NL	54%	62%	27%	32%
** Pregnant	53%	69%	32%	42%

* NP-NL= non-pregnant, non-lactating
** Cut-off point for anaemia is < 12 g/100 ml for all except
for pregnant women (< 11 g/100 ml)

The surveys in East Java were conducted two decades ago. It is, however, very probable that the nutritional status of adolescents has not changed much between the late 1970s and the 1990s, as is the case for preschool children and women of reproductive age (Kardjati 1992; Kodiat 1994). One may conclude that the nutritional stress during reproduction is superimposed on the poor nutritional status during adolescence and early childhood.

Safe motherhood: issues and options

In industrial countries the health and nutritional status of the population improved over a period of one or two centuries – at the same pace as the level of education, buying power, knowledge, availability of health services and biomedical technology. Each decade the survivors were healthier and better nourished. With the improvement of education, health and nutrition became a felt need, people became aware of their entitlements and through a democratic political system obtained the power to claim their rights. Maternal mortality decreased as a result of better health and nutrition throughout a woman's life cycle (secular trend in height), improvement of environmental hygiene, the increased availability and utilization of adequate obstetric and postnatal care. Sexual and reproductive health according to the present definition (the individual right to determine ...) followed the emphasis on women as mothers.

In developing countries the main achievement of the health sector in the past 50 years is the significant reduction in infant mortality (consequently an increase in life expectancy) and to a lesser extent in child (under-five) mortality. This achievement is mainly attributable to *magic bullets*, such as immunization. With environmental sanitation, food availability and education lagging behind, the surviving children are not healthy and well-nourished. The meagre gains in relative reduction in malnutrition (a decrease in the prevalence of underweight in preschool children of 2-3% per year) has only statistical significance as the absolute numbers of nutritionally deprived increase by millions each year (SCN News 1995). It is not surprising that no spectacular decline in maternal mortality has been attained. No magic bullets exist to address maternal morbidity and mortality. As underdeveloped children become stunted adults with impaired functional performance, each next generation will have larger numbers of women at risk of dying as a consequence of reproduction.

During the Population and Family Planning Conference, Bucharest, 1974, and the First World Food Conference, Rome, 1974, the main concern was rapid population growth and the limits of economic growth and food production. The introduced family planning programmes were largely driven by this demographic motive. Little account was taken of the social, cultural and personal realities of reproductive life.

The increasing evidence of the disproportionately high maternal mortality rate resulted in the Safe Motherhood Initiative at a conference in Nairobi in 1987, which has been adopted by most developing countries (Herz & Measham 1987). To reach the goal of reducing maternal illness and death by half by the year 2000, the World Bank, the World Health Organization and the United Nations Agency for Population Activities launched 'a short-term strategy that would make family planning services and maternal health care more effective – by improving quality, increasing access and educating the public about the importance of such services and how they can best be used' (Maine 1991: 19; Tinker & Koblinsky 1993: 10). While acknowledging the significant contribution of poor nutrition to maternal mortality, only the distribution of iron pills were included in the recommendations for the essential services for women (Tinker et al. 1994; World Bank 1993). The

International Conference on Population and Development, Cairo, 1994, and the Fourth World Conference on Women, Beijing, 1995, broadened the focus to include sexual health and reproductive rights of couples. It should, however, be realized that women's entitlement to basic needs, such as food, must be recognized by the society and couples first before sexual and reproductive rights can be addressed.

As far as health service delivery is concerned, the evolution was from Maternal and Child Health (MCH) care in the 1950s-60s with separate antenatal and well-baby clinics to supposedly comprehensive Primary Health Care (PHC) in the late 1970s to mid-1980s – which broke down to selective and fragmented PHC. Maternal health in PHC was reduced to training traditional birth attendants and the distribution of delivery kits. UNICEF promoted and supported the Child Survival and Development (CSD) strategy with a focus on growth monitoring, oral rehydration, breast feeding promotion and immunizations (GOBI). The broader and relevant GOBI-FFF strategy (family planning, food supplementation and female education) did not materialize, for unreported reasons. WHO concentrated on the Essential Drugs Programme (EDP), the control of diarrhoeal diseases (CDD) and lately the management of acute respiratory infections (ARI).

In the conventional direct nutrition interventions, usually the responsibility of the Ministry of Health, women have been over-targeted rather than under-targeted. However, there is an important difference between being the intended target and being the beneficiary of an intervention. The nutrition interventions were primarily designed to reduce malnutrition among children. Programs in the field of rural development, agriculture and income generation aim at food security of the family. They seldom take into account that a disproportionate burden of the extra inputs are shouldered by women. The higher work load, and thus energy expenditure, may be detrimental to women's health and nutrition. Although family food security is a prerequisite for nutrition security for all its members, maternal nutrition is ultimately determined by access to and control of available resources. The Agenda following the International Nutrition Conference in Adelaide, 1992 reiterates pledges to achieve food and nutrition security (FAO/WHO 1992; WHO 1995) but lacks innovative and creative plans to address women's nutrition security.

Somehow, the policy debate in the 1990s has not resulted in realistic intervention approaches which take the development levels of the countries concerned into account. To assess which direct interventions are relevant, feasible and cost-effective for safe motherhood, this is defined as:

a woman's health and nutritional status which ensures maternal and infant outcomes of pregnancy with minimal risks of mortality, maternal depletion and growth failure in infancy. The definition excludes the social dimensions of women's health and the gender perspective of reproductive health as they go beyond the topic of this paper. However, the definition is broader than the current approach of the Safe Motherhood Initiative which concentrates on family planning, obstetric care, abortions and sexually transmitted diseases, HIV/AIDS.

Setting priorities

Need always exceeds resources, and location-specific programmes are required to increase cost-effectiveness while maintaining the guiding principle of equity. Priority setting starts with an assessment of needs and demands which require a gender-differentiated health information system. At no extra cost, health professionals can tally available information on morbidities and health service utilization by males and females. Similarly, a participatory appraisal of the local health situation by gender should be part of the training package of village health and development workers and traditional birth attendants. It is generally accepted that the (UNICEF) triple A principle (assessment, analysis, action) should govern the selection of essential interventions which are understood and endorsed by all actors. A great deal of emphasis is given to community participation in PHC, nutrition programmes, and recently the SMI. In fact, donor bias usually dominates the type of interventions selected, and line agencies such as the Ministries of Health concentrate on provision of the services implied. The community, families and women are seldom involved in the decision-making process. Their participation is only encouraged during the implementation of predetermined programmes. The emphasis is on securing consensus for these activities, rather than encouraging initiatives originating from the community. Unless families/women's priorities are taken into consideration, culture-sensitive approaches to empowerment adhered to and the role of different actors (government, NGOs, the community, families and women) jointly agreed upon, valuable resources and time will be wasted.

Cost-effective obstetric care

About 36% of life-years of women of reproductive age (WRA) are lost due to reproductive health problems. By contrast, the equivalent figure for men is 12%. Emergency obstetric care (EOC) was introduced to ensure adequate services for risk pregnancies and deliveries on time (WHO 1994). While conceptually correct, it may not be feasible universally. Like any intervention, the effectiveness of EOC is highly sensitive to its environment, such as population density, the road infrastructure, the existing structure of health services, the number of trained human resources relative to tasks, to name a few. In addition, screening for complications is ineffective as a measure to reduce MMR as there are often no early warning signals that an emergency complication is likely to occur (Maine 1991; UNICEF 1996). The following considerations will show that EOC is only a cost-effective intervention in areas of high population density, i.e. urban communities.

The availability of skilled professionals is essential, but trained medical doctors and midwives need to attend enough complicated cases to retain their skills, and they should be accessible when needed. Let us assume that a medical doctor (MD) must attend 2 cases per week to remain skilled, i.e. 104 cases per year. For a population with a crude birth rate (CBR) of 45/1000 population (1990 average for Africa), in which 20% of pregnancies are complicated (estimate based on data of Koblinsky et al. 1995), EOC will be relevant if one MD covers a population of 11,500 people (5x104= 520 deliveries; 520: 45= 11,500 population). To be effective, EOC should be reachable within one hour, which is rarely the case in rural areas. The option of having pregnant women at risk admitted a few weeks before the expected date of delivery entails too many logistic problems from the provider as well as client side.

Indonesia has decided (at the recommendation of the World Bank) to post one midwife in isolated villages, mainly in the outer islands. So far, this component of SMI faces many problems (MotherCare Indonesia 1997). To meet the need for about 50,000 midwives in one Five-Year Plan period, the training was reduced from 4 to 2 years. As a result, the so-called village midwives were insufficiently skilled and lacked self-confidence. The degree of social acceptance of village midwives was not as desired by the programme implementors (Ministry of Health). The village community was supposed to co-finance the maternity-cum-house for the midwife. However, they were too poor to do so or for some other reasons failed to respond. The midwife was not trained and not allowed to give curative care, which further undermined her status. Supposedly she had access to the pregnant women, but in reality this was not the case. In the provinces outside Java and Bali, the population density is low, the terrain rough or mountainous and the roads not passable in the rainy season, certainly for women in advanced pregnancy. Even if all pregnant women would avail themselves of the midwife's services, this type of EOC will turn out to be not affordable nor a cost-effective approach to reduce maternal mortality. Take as an example a village size of 1000 population (quite realistic in the geographical areas concerned), a CBR of 30 per 1000 population and a MMR of 4/1000 deliveries (average for Indonesia in the 1990s). It will take 1000: 30= about 33 years for the village midwife to encounter 4 maternal deaths. She may have prevented 2 of them (she can't intervene surgically or provide blood transfusions). With a monthly salary of USD 135 the 2 maternal deaths would have been avoided at a cost of about USD 53,460 (33x12 months times USD135) for salary alone!

Nutrition as part of the essential package of SMI

Effective reproductive health programs could alleviate only about one-third of the burden of disease among women of reproductive age (Turmen 1995). It is unknown to what degree poor maternal nutrition is an underlying or contributory factor to maternal and infant mortality. The World Bank and the WHO introduced in 1993 a measure of the global burden of disease by combining (a) losses from premature death and (b) loss of healthy life resulting from disability. The unit used was termed disability-adjusted life-years or DALYs (World Bank 1993: 25). Overall the burden of malnutrition and the micronutrient deficiencies contribute 33% to DALYs in sub-Saharan Africa, 22% in the Indian subcontinent and 16% in Southeast Asia (Murray & Lopez 1996: 312). Based on the magnitude of nutritional deficiencies among women of reproductive age and the relation with the major causes of maternal deaths, as discussed earlier, a conservative estimate would be that this non-infectious morbidity accounts for 25% of MMR.

Unfortunately, health information systems only differentiate women when they are pregnant and nutritional indicators are seldom included. The BMI is not yet a commonly applied indicator of nutritional risk among women, although weight and height are measured at antenatal clinics and easy applicable nomograms are available. For reasons stated earlier, pre-pregnant weight is an important indicator of safe motherhood (risk level 45 kg in African communities and 42 kg in Asian/Latin American communities). Outside health institutions the (left) mid-upper arm circumference can replace BMI, and the risk cut-off is 22.5 cm, irrespective of her physiological state (pregnant, lactating or non-pregnant/non-lactating). The East Java data strongly suggest that a CED prevalence among women of reproductive age above 20% is associated with poor outcomes of pregnancy of public health magnitude which warrants dietary intervention as part of a safe motherhood program.

Nutrition interventions for women of reproductive age are generally considered (too) expensive. Food supplementation for pregnant women costs about USD 23.65 per DALY. It compares favourably with the cost of Expanded Program of Immunizations for under-fives which amounts to USD 13.2 per beneficiary and USD 20-34 per DALY or with food supplementation for preschool children which costs USD 62.65 per DALY (Pinstrup-Andersen et al. 1993). Micronutrient supplementation is the cheapest and the most cost-effective. The price for iron supplementation to pregnant women is USD 12.80 per DALY (Levin et al. 1993). The choice of interventions depends on the most important nutritional deficiencies prevailing in an area and the resources available.

No information is available for nutrition expenditures by the public sector, but most likely it does not exceed 3% of the government's health budget (Himes 1995). Only 9% of external assistance to the health sector in 1990 was earmarked for nutrition (Murray & Lopez 1994). Hence, nutrition is accorded modest financial resources, operational and otherwise compared with the magnitude of the problem. Unfortunately, there is little evidence of restructuring aid in support of health and nutrition goals. Instead, a fall in overall aid levels was observed in 1993 compared with 1990 (UNICEF 1995). The 20/20 Initiative, formulated by five UN organizations and presented at the Social Summit in Copenhagen in 1994, offers an opportunity for more adequate funding for social services from national and international sources. The Initiative suggested that financial allocations to such services be increased to 20% of the total government budget, which will be complemented by 20% of donor development assistance (UNDP et al. 1994; UNCTAD et al. 1996). If properly targeted, this additional budget can substantially meet short-term basic social needs, reduce the worst aspects of poverty and pave the way for the achievement of longer term human development objectives. Nevertheless, the resources will not be sufficient to cover all basic needs. The affordability and sustainability of food supplementation or food rations are enhanced if the safe motherhood programme is packaged into comprehensive PHC, livelihood programs of the agricultural sector or micro-credit programmes, as exemplified by the Grameen Bank in Bangladesh.

Adolescents as an entry point for safe motherhood

Reproductive health is an outcome of past health, and it sets the stage for the health of the next generation. Nutrition is important at all ages, so that the woman enters childbearing age with normal height, weight, pelvic size and nutritional status. In most developing countries adolescent girls are at greater risk of undernutrition than boys because girls are engaged in heavy household work and economically productive activities from early life without increased food intake. In the health sector adolescents fall through the cracks. School health services, if any, have primary school children as their target group. The narrow focus of SMI is illustrated by its attention on adolescents within the boundaries of pregnancy-and sex-related problems.

Adolescents, in particular girls, are a relevant target group for interventions because the prevalence of CED and micronutrient deficiencies are already high in the period immediately preceding reproductive life. It is more rational to intervene before they start to bear and nurture children as supplementation during pregnancy can hardly overcome the pre-existing nutritional deficiencies in the short time of 3-4 months. Moreover, it is more feasible to intervene during adolescence. There are fewer cultural constraints and food taboos than during pregnancy. Adolescence is also a period of great opportunity for preparing girls and boys to become productive and confident adults with proper health and nutrition behaviours. They can be a target group as well as agents of change. Investing in youth is investing in the future (Kurz et al. 1994). It may in the long term turn out to be the most cost-effective health intervention, imitating the evolution of health and nutrition in industrialized countries. The education sector offers a window of opportunity to reach the school-age population. Even in countries where school enrolment for girls is low, it far exceeds the coverage of obstetric care, particularly in rural areas. The longer and regular exposure to nutrition and health education and dietary intervention in schools may shorten the time frame for a positive change in dietary behaviour, thus enhancing the sustainability of any intervention. Examples of increased attention for nutritional health in adolescents from Indonesia are: micronutrient supplementation to factory and plantation workers (usually young girls), nutrition education and dietary improvement in Moslem boarding schools, attended by children, 12-17 years of age, in preparation for marital life (*pondok pesantren*).

Closing remarks

There are no short-cuts to reducing maternal mortality. Over the past decades women's health policies were driven by fertility regulation, followed by medical interventions for safe motherhood with a focus on obstetric service delivery and lately, as the HIV/AIDS epidemic emerged, to sexually transmitted infections and culminating in the current policy for sexual and reproductive health. While these strategies will be eminently beneficial to women, in the short term they will not reap any benefits unless women's entitlement to food and other basic needs is strongly promoted and acknowledged through an adequate financial allocation.

Packaging of interventions is potentially the most cost-effective. The fragmentation of health programmes has been a counter-productive evolution in health care. It is time to address women's health throughout the life cycle and within the context of family health.

It should, however, be realized that poor health and nutritional status of women are also noted in communities where the availability of food and health services are not major constraints. Promotion of women's access to and control of resources are beyond what is commonly understood as health interventions. Yet, the health sector can serve as a catalyst and facilitator. By including the economic dimensions of women's health in policy debates and grassroot level group discussions, the health worker can make actors aware that investments in girls and women's nutrition and health have high returns in productivity, educationability and the quality of life of the next generation.

Similarly, the health sector can take a lead role in integrating women's health and nutrition into rural development activities and income-generating activities. Ironically, other sectors have been more considerate in these efforts, as illustrated by the Grameen Bank in Bangladesh or the Women's World Banking Association.

What is required for women's health reform is a fruitful merging of creative technological interventions, the conviction that it can be done and the political will.

Notes

1   The first report on a direct link between micronutrient deficiencies and maternal mortality was presented at the annual meeting of the International Vitamin A

Consultative Group in Cairo, September 1997. The preliminary result of the study providing an oral weekly dose of vitamin A to 20,000 married Nepalese women was a decrease in pregnancy-related mortality by a remarkable 45% (Keith West, Johns Hopkins in collaboration with Netra Jyoti Sangh, personal communication).

2 A comprehensive overview of the studies was presented as a monograph (Kusin & Kardjati 1994).

Literature

Anersson, R. & S. Bergstrom

1997 'Maternal nutrition and socio-economic status as determinants of birth-weight in chronically malnourished African women.' *Trop Med Intern Health* 2: 1080-1087.

Barker, D.J.P. (ed.)

1992 *Fetal and infant origins of adult disease.* London: British Medical Journal-Publishing Group.

Bucher, H.C., R.J. Cook, G.H. Guyatt et al.

1996a 'Effects of a dietary calcium supplementation on blood pressure: A meta-analysis of randomized controlled trials.' *JAMA* 275: 1006-1012.

Bucher, H.C., R.J. Cook, G.H. Guyatt et al.

1996b 'Effect of calcium supplementation on pregnancy-induced hypertension and eclampsia: A meta-analysis of randomized controlled trials.' *JAMA* 275: 1113-1117.

Dibley, M.J., J.B. Goldsby, M.W. Staehling & F.L. Trowbridge

1987 'Development of normalised growth curves for the international growth reference.' *Am J Clin Nutr* 46: 736-48.

FAO/WHO

1992 *Final Report of the International Conference on Nutrition.* Rome: FAO.

Herz, B. & A.R. Measham

1987 *The Safe Motherhood Initiative. Proposals for Action.* World Bank Discussion Papers No.9. Washington: World Bank.

Himes, J.R. (ed)

1995 *Implementing the Convention on the Rights of the Child. Resource mobilization in low-income countries.* The Hague: Martinus Nijhof Publishers.

Hutter, I.

1994 *Being pregnant in rural South India. Nutrition of women and well-being of children.* PhD Thesis, Groningen University.

James, W.P.T, A. Ferro-Luzzi & J.C. Waterlow
   1988   'Definition of chronic energy deficiency in adults.' *Eur J Clin Nutr* 42: 969-982.

Koblinsky, M., O.M.R. Campbell & S.D. Harlow
   1995   'Mother and more: A broader perspective on women's health.' In: M. Koblinsky, J. Timyan & J. Gay (eds), *The health of women: A global perspective*. San Francisco: Westview Press, pp. 33-61.

Kodiat, B.A.
   1994   *Nutrition in Indonesia: Problems, trends, strategy and programs*. Jakarta: MOH.

Kolsteren, P.W.
   1996   'Growth faltering in Madura, Indonesia. A comparison with the NCHS reference and data from Kasongo, Zaire.' *Ann Trop Paediatr* 16: 233-242.

Kurz, K.M. & C. Johnson-Welch
   1994   *The nutrition and lives of adolescents in developing countries*. Washington: International Center for Research on Women.

Kusin, J.A., W.M. Van Steenbergen, S.A. Lakhani, A.A.J. Jansen & U.H. Renqvist
   1984   'Food consumption in pregnancy and lactation.' In: J.K. van Ginneken & A.S. Muller (eds), *Maternal and Child Health in Rural Kenya*. London: Croom Helm, pp. 127-142.

Kusin, J.A. & A.A.J. Jansen
   1986   'Maternal nutrition and birth weight: A selective review and some observations in Machakos, Kenya.' *Ann Trop Pediat* 6: 3-9.

Kusin, J.A. & S. Kardjati
   1994   *Maternal and Child Nutrition in Madura, Indonesia*. Amsterdam: Koninklijk Instituut voor de Tropen.

Kusin, J.A., S. Kardjati & U.H. Renqvist
   1994   'Maternal Body Mass Index: The functional significance during reproduction.' *Eur J Clin Nutr* 48, suppl.3: s56-s67.

Leslie, J.
   1994   'Improving the nutrition of women in the Third World.' In: P. Pinstrup-Andersen, D. Pelletier & H. Alderman (eds), *Child growth and nutrition in developing countries: Priorities for action*. Ithaca NY: Cornell University Press, pp. 117-138.

Levin, H.M., E. Pollitt, R. Galloway & J. McGuire
   1993   'Micronutrient Deficiency Disorders.' In: D.T. Jamison, W.H. Mosley, A.R. Measham & J.L. Bobadilla (eds), *Disease priorities in developing countries*. Oxford: OUP, pp. 421-451.

Maine, D.
   1991   *Safe Motherhood programs: Options and issues*. New York: Columbia University, Center for Population and Family Health.

Martyn, C.N., D.J.P. Barker & C. Osmond
   1996   'Mother's pelvic size, fetal growth and death from stroke and coronary
           heart disease in men in the UK.' *Lancet* 348: 1264-68.
McGuire, J. & B.M. Popkin
   1989   'Beating the zero-sum game: Women and nutrition in the Third World.'
           Food Nutr Bull 11: 38-63.
Merchant, K., R. Martorell & J. Haas
   1990   'Consequences for maternal nutrition of reproductive stress across con-
           secutive pregnancies.' *Am J Clin Nutr* 52: 616-620.
MotherCare/Indonesia
   1997   Vol.6, no.4, Arlington VA: John Snow.
Murray, C.J.L. & A.D. Lopez
   1994   *Global comparative assessments in the health sector. Disease burden, ex-
           penditures and intervention packages.* Geneva: WHO.
Murray, C.J.L. & A.D. Lopez
   1996   *The Global Burden of Disease. A comprehensive assessment of mortality
           and disability from diseases, injuries and risk factors in 1990 and projected
           to 2020.* Geneva: WHO.
Norton, R.
   1994   'Maternal nutrition during pregnancy as it affects infant growth, develop-
           ment and health.' *SCN News* 11: 10-14.
Pinstrup-Andersen, P., S. Burger, J.P. Habicht & K. Petersen
   1993   'Protein-energy malnutrition.' In: D.T. Jamison, W.H. Mosley, A.R.
           Measham & J.L. Bobadilla (eds), *Disease priorities in developing countries.*
           Oxford: OUP, pp. 391-412.
Pitkin, R. (ed.)
   1990   *Nutrition during pregnancy.* Washington DC: National Academic Press,
           pp. 222-236.
Prentice, A.M., G.R. Goldberg & A. Prentice
   1994   'Body Mass Index and lactation performance.' *Eur J Clin Nutr* 48, suppl.
           3: s78-s89.
Subcommittee on Nutrition
   1995   'Update on the nutrition nituation.' *SCN News* 12. *Geneva:* WHO.
Stein, C.E., C.H.D. Fall, K. Kumaran, C. Osmond, V., Cox & D.J.P. Barker
   1996   'Fetal growth and coronary heart disease in South India.' *Lancet* 348:
           1269-73.
Tinker, A. & M.A. Koblinsky
   1993   *Making Motherhood Safe.* World Bank Discussion Papers No. 202.
           Washington: World Bank.
Tinker, A., P. Daly, C. Green, H. Saxenian, R. Lashminarayanan & K. Gill
   1994   *Women's health and nutrition.* World Bank Discussion Papers No. 256.
           Washington: World Bank.

Turmen, T.

1995 *Reproductive Health: From rhetoric to reality.* Paper presented at the European Conference on Tropical Medicine. Hamburg, 23 October 1995.

UNDP, UNESCO, UNFPA, UNICEF, WHO

1994 *The 20/20 Initiative. Achieving universal access to basic social services for sustainable human development.* A note prepared jointly for the 20/20 Meeting, December 1994, Oslo.

UNCTAD, UNDP, UNFPA, UNICEF

1996 *Implementing the 20/20 Initiative: Issues regarding definitions, modalities and monitoring.* Paper prepared in consultation with representatives of Bangladesh, Canada, Chile, France, the Netherlands, Norway, Uganda and the World Bank, and presented at the 20/20 Meeting, April 1996, Oslo.

UNDP

1996 *Human Development Report 1995* Oxford: OUP.

UNICEF

1995 *The State of the World's Children 1995.* New York: UNICEF.

1996 *The Progress of Nations.* New York: UNICEF.

1997 *The State of the World's Children 1997.* New York: UNICEF.

WHO

1990 *WHO approaches to health in adolescence. Division of Family Health.* Geneva: WHO.

1994 *Mother-Baby Package: Implementing safe motherhood in countries.* Division of Family Health. Geneva: WHO.

1995 *Nutrition. Highlights of recent activities in the context of the World Declaration and Plan of Action for Nutrition.* Geneva: WHO.

1996 *Fact Sheet.* No. 119. Geneva: WHO.

WHO/UNICEF

1996 *Revised estimates of maternal mortality: A new approach by WHO and UNICEF.* Geneva: WHO.World Bank

1993 *World Development Report 1993. Investing in Health.* Washington: World Bank.

CHAPTER VI

Contextualizing Reproductive Health Care[1]

ANITA HARDON

In 1978, at the International Conference on Primary Health Care in Alma Ata, the world health community adopted primary health care (PHC) as a concept and as a strategy that would address inequality in the health status of people in developed and developing countries, and within countries. PHC was defined as essential health care, based on practical, scientifically sound, and socially acceptable technology made universally available to individuals and families in the community through their full participation and at a cost that the community and country could afford. Health was defined as a state of complete physical, mental and social well-being, not merely the absence of disease (WHO/UNICEF 1978). Eight components of PHC were defined, among which was maternal and child care, including family planning.

Sixteen years after Alma Ata, at the International Conference on Population and Development (ICPD) in Cairo in September 1994, the international health community adopted another new health concept: reproductive health. The definition of reproductive health, included in paragraph 7.2 of the final document of the ICPD (Alcala 1994) reads as follows: 'Reproductive health is a state of complete physical, mental and social well-being and not merely the absence of disease or infirmity, in all matters relating to the reproductive system and to its functions and processes. Reproductive health therefore implies that people are able to have a satisfying and safe sex life and that they have the capability to reproduce and the freedom to decide if, when and how often to do so.'

The reproductive health concept emerged partly in response to the critique of women's health advocates on the implementation of family planning and maternal and child care components of PHC. Family planning, according to the critics, had focussed too much on achieving demographic goals, i.e. fertility decline. Also, maternal and child care services were seen to perpetuate existing gender inequalities by approaching women either as mothers or as married women, ignoring unmarried women and non-mothers (Germain & Ordway 1989). Overall, PHC programmes had emphasized services for the sick child, immunization, and the prevention of maternal mortality, ignoring other gynaecological, mental and emotional problems of women related to their reproductive health. The reproductive health care approach ideally would address this imbalance.

Of all PHC components, family planning had in the 1980s and 1990s become the most accessible health service worldwide. This was mainly because of the perceived need of population planners to decrease fertility rates and reduce population growth and the related donor funding for the distribution of contraceptives. The critique of women's health advocates on the conduct of family planning programs coincided with the observation of population planners and family planning programme administrators that the distribution of contraceptives alone was not sufficient to produce fertility decline. High percentages of women were found to discontinue contraceptive use, and a large unmet need for family planning services was observed. It was realized that the quality of care would need to be improved to enhance continued contraceptive use (Jain 1992). Improved quality of care would include more attention for women's health.

The emergence of the reproductive health concept can, finally, also be related to the HIV/AIDS epidemic. The increased distribution of condoms for HIV/AIDS control affected family planning programs which distributed the same methods for contraceptive purposes. International health planners recognized that HIV/AIDS control could be strengthened if existing family planning services were broadened to include the promotion of condoms not only as contraceptive but also as protection against the transmission of sexually transmitted diseases, including HIV.

In the wake of the Cairo conference, estimates have been made of the burden of reproductive health problems worldwide. Table 1 gives the magnitude of the most common reproductive health problems, as estimated by the World Health Organization (WHO 1997).

One can imagine that implementation of reproductive health care to deal with all these health problems requires a revolution in health care. It requires family planning and health administrators to plan jointly the implementation of the programmes and to define cost-effective packages of good-quality integrated services shaped to the specific needs of diverse clients in different settings and available to all who need them (Aitken & Reichenbach 1994).

Table 1 Selected aspects of reproductive ill health, 1990-1995, as estimated by the WHO (1997)

Category	Women	Men	Worldwide
Maternal death annually	585 thousand		585 thousand
Cases of severe maternal morbidity	20 million		20 million
Perinatal deaths annually			7.6 million
Unsafe abortions annually	20 million		20 million
Adults living with HIV/AIDS	9 million	13 million	22 million
Cases of curable STDs annually	166 million	167 million	333 million
Prevalence of STDs	175 million	75 million	250 million
Infertile couples			60-80 million
Women living with invasive cervical cancers	2 million		2 million
New cases of cervical cancer annually	450 thousand		450 thousand
Women with genital mutilation	85-110 million		85-110 million
Couples with unmet family planning needs			120 million

Priorities and processes

There are two problems with the new integrated reproductive health concept that need to be considered. The first is that the concept is not accompanied by a strategy, as was the PHC concept accepted in Alma Ata. Secondly, there is no clarity on the way in which priorities should be set. Is the implementation of reproductive health care to be top-down; or are we calling for a participatory approach, including action research to determine people's needs and concerns, as was advocated in the Alma Ata document on primary health care?

With respect to the priorities, the main question is how and who is to set them. There is an increasing tendency to base priorities on cost-effectiveness analysis done at the national and international level of health care. The World Bank, following a cost-effectiveness approach, has defined priorities which if followed lead to a shortlist of programme components. The 1993 World Development Report, which had as its leading theme *Investing in Health*, lists AIDS prevention as a priority public health intervention along with services to ensure pregnancy-related (prenatal, childbirth and postpartum) care, in order to prevent the almost half a million maternal deaths that occur each year in developing countries. Other priorities are family planning services (improved access to these services could save as many as 850,000 children from dying each year and eliminate as many as 100,000 of the maternal deaths that occur annually) and control of STDs, which account for more than 250 million new cases of debilitating and sometimes fatal diseases each year. The World Bank considers these clinical interventions as highly cost-effective, often costing substantially less than 50 USD per disability-adjusted life-year (DALY) gained. Treatment of infertility, the provision of safe abortion, and the treatment of other reproductive morbidities such as cervical cancer are not listed in the limited list of essential services, and if the World Bank planning strategy is followed, they would not be included in the government-provided health programmes. But who is to decide on such issues of priorities? Should it be based on cost-effectiveness analysis, or rather on the definition of priorities by the target groups through processes of needs assessment and community participation?

Reproductive health as a gender issue

Women suffer more from reproductive health problems than men. The *Investing in Health* report cited above found that in women of reproductive age in developing countries, reproductive ill health accounts for 36% of the total disease burden, compared with 12% for men (World Bank 1993). Sex differentials in incidence and prevalence of reproductive health problems are affected by the value system in societies that gives indications for the ideal behaviour of men and women and determines their different social roles and statuses (Appelman & Reysoo 1994). In most societies women are seen to be subservient to men. They primarily gain status by having children and caring for their families. Gender inequalities adversely affect reproductive health problems such as the incidence of unwanted pregnancy, the unmet need for contraception, the lack of access to antenatal care and the risks of maternal mortality.

Gender and Reproductive Health research

The collaborative research project *Gender, reproductive health and population policies* (GRHPP) aims at generating more innovative knowledge about women's and men's experiences with and perspectives on fertility regulation technologies and services in diverse socio-cultural settings.[2] This innovative action-research project was formulated in the early 1990s (long before Cairo) in response to (a) critiques of the conduct on demographically driven family planning programs in developing countries and (b) concern about the introduction of longer-acting, provider-dependent contraceptives to achieve fertility decline. There was a clear need for systematic research, emphasizing the views and experiences of people who use fertility regulation services and technologies. Based on the results of the studies, the researchers aim to contribute to more need-oriented and gender-sensitive development interventions in the field of reproductive health.[3]

In this contribution, I will present findings from two country studies (the Philippines and Mozambique) that focus on fertility regulation, and I will outline the policy recommendations that can be formulated based on the empirical findings. In doing so, I intend to show how reproductive health problems at the local level can be adapted to meet people's concerns and needs for fertility regulation services.

Contextualizing fertility regulation

The 1994 Cairo conference (ICPD) reached a consensus that reproductive health implies that people are able to have a satisfying and safe sex life and that they have the capability to reproduce and the freedom to decide if, when and how often to do so. To achieve this ideal, men and women need to be informed and to have access to safe, effective, affordable and acceptable methods of family planning of their choice (Alcala 1994).

People's use of contraceptives has been studied extensively in order to evaluate the coverage of family planning programs and to determine barriers to contraceptive use. The underlying assumption of many studies is: the higher the contraceptive prevalence, the better. The studies tend to have a narrow focus, describing what people know about modern contraceptives, what their attitudes are towards these methods, and to what extent they actually use them, divorced from the other social and economical realities of their lives. The adoption of a modern innovation – contraception – through diffusion is presented as the determinant of fertility decline (Greenhalgh 1995). In such contraception studies culture tends to be treated as something separate from the rest of social life, as something that facilitates or obstructs contraceptive communication. They usually result in recommendations on how cultural barriers can be overcome.

The studies in the GRHPP project have a different perspective and approach. Fertility regulation is situated in the lives of women and men. Unlike conventional studies on fertility regulation, the focus is not on current users of specific methods. By interviewing women about their reproductive life histories, the researchers uncover how they use different methods at different points in their reproductive lives. The studies show how women go through phases of wanting to be pregnant, conceiving or not conceiving, not wanting to be pregnant but wanting to have more children later, using fertility regulation methods, not using fertility regulation methods because of perceived side effects, becoming pregnant and having an abortion, and so on.

This implies that we should not only look into issues of fertility control, but also into issues related to perceived infertility. Infertility is an issue that has received very little attention in the international health policy arena. The ICPD does recognize infertility as a problem, recommending prevention of infertility and appropriate treatment where feasible. In practice, however, infertility prevention and treatment are rarely included in reproductive and primary health programmes. It is, for example, not proposed as a priority public health intervention in the World Bank's *Investing in Health* report, despite the fact that an estimated 60-80 million couples experience unwanted infertility, a figure which is nearly equal to the estimated yearly burden of unwanted pregnancies (Aitken & Reichenbach 1994).

Very little research has been done to describe the problem of infertility from the perspective of the people suffering from the condition. In the GRHPP project a number of studies focus on infertility in order to elucidate women's and men's experiences with the problem in diverse sociocultural contexts.

STDs, primarily gonorrhoea and genital *Chlamydia* infection, are one of the main causes of infertility. Among selected populations in sub-Saharan Africa, STD-induced infertility is estimated to affect as many as one-third to one-half of all couples (WHO 1987).

Few studies on people's experiences with infertility exist. In one of the rare examples, Inhorn (1994) describes how among the urban and rural poor in Egypt, female infertility is often attributed to *Kabsa*, a form of 'boundary crossing' by symbolically polluted individuals into the rooms of reproductively vulnerable women. According to widely accepted normative standards, women reproductively 'bound' by *Kabsa* must overcome its effects or be barred from achieving normal adult personhood. Women bear the major burden of infertility in terms of blame, social ostracism, and the relentless search for therapies which often prove torturous and even harmful.

Fertility regulation in urban poor communities in the Philippines

Let us now move towards a local sociocultural setting in the Philippines, to understand fertility regulation in context.[4] The main question that emerges from the results of fieldwork in Metro Manila is: why do women in urban poor communities in the Philippines resort to abortion methods regularly, instead of using the modern contraceptives that are accessible in the communities to control their fertility?

The most recent (1993) national demographic survey (NDS) shows that knowledge of contraception is extremely high in the Philippines (96% of married women knew about contraceptive pills and 92% about sterilization), while only 25% of currently married women of reproductive age are using modern methods of family planning (nearly half of these 'users' are sterilized, around one-third use the Pill, and the rest use IUDs and condoms). A large percentage (60%) of married women of reproductive age do not use modern contraceptives, while only 9% say that they want a child in the coming 2 years.

Family planning services are mostly provided by the government rather than by NGOs or the private sector in the Philippines. The NDS calculated that around three-fourths of women using modern contraception had received their contraceptive at a government hospital or clinic. That these services are available is not always clear to women. The NDS found that 37% of married women of reproductive age were not aware where they could obtain the contraceptive pill.

The government family planning services has been in existence since the early 1970s, when the Philippine population policy was supported, and the programme was funded by USAID. In the Marcos days the programme was not noted for its efficiency, though no formal evaluation was done. When

Cory Aquino, a devout Catholic, came to power, the Catholic bishops opposed the programme more vocally, which led to considerable public controversy about the programme and a near standstill of its implementation. USAID in fact pulled out in 1989 because of the slow implementation. Ties with the international donors were renewed in 1992 when Fidel Ramos became president, and the programme, was revitalized under the leadership of health secretary Flavier. The plan to reinforce the dormant programme led to fierce attacks from conservative Catholic groups such as Opus Dei and Pro-life. The Catholic Church promotes natural family planning methods, such as the *Billings* method, which rely on abstinence during the fertile period of a woman.

In the urban poor communities in Manila, contraceptives, particularly the contraceptive pill, are easily accessible in government health centres and over the counter in pharmacies. In some communities church-run community-based health programmes promote natural family planning methods.

People in the urban poor communities are motivated to limit their family size. In the harsh urban poor environment, having children costs money for schooling and food and time of parents that otherwise could be spent on income-earning. Many urban poor families lack extended family support for childcare while parents work.

The contraceptive pill is in fact the most accessible and most used method of contraception in the urban poor communities. In my own study among urban poor in Manila, among a sample of 137 women with pre-school children in 1987, around one-fourth was using the contraceptive pill, another 15% were using IUD and only 11% condoms. No one at the time was using injectables (Hardon 1991).

Perceptions about how the Pill works vary in the urban poor communities. Some women stress that it kills sperm. Others say it goes to the uterus and acts as a barrier. Many know the fixed regime explained in the family planning clinics: it should be started on the fifth day of menstruation and taken daily. A positive attribute of the Pill in the view of many women is that it makes you fat (*mataba*) if the pill is *hiyang* (suitable for the person taking the pill). If the pill is not *hiyang*, then you lose your appetite and become thin.

Women in the urban poor communities feel ambivalent about the Pill. They value its contraceptive effects, but fear its adverse affects. A very common notion is that the pills that are taken daily accumulate in the uterus, thus causing *kanser*, as one woman expressed to a researcher in Tondo (Manila):

When you take too much, there will be a stock in the *matres* (uterus), a mass, that can lead to *kanser*.

Having less menstruation is an effect that is said to aggravate the ill effects, because the uterus is then not cleaned properly. Women believe that a good menstrual flow cleans the body of dirt. The accumulation of pills in the uterus is also said to lead to infections. *Cleanups* are also needed to prevent such infections.

Another effect that is commonly attributed to the Pill is *init ng ulo*, irritability (literal translation: hotheaded). *Init ng ulo* is also related to the changes in menstruation caused by the Pill. If menstruation is scarce, not only dirt but also heat accumulates in the body (Tan 1987).

Because of the perceived adverse effects of the Pill and other contraceptives, women tend to use the methods only for short periods of time. Not surprisingly, unwanted pregnancies occur often. When this is the case, women resort to abortions, despite the fact that abortion is illegal in the Philippines. Abortions are very common in urban poor communities. Jocano (1975) in an extensive study of an urban slum (with an estimated population of 1000 people of 20 years and above) recorded 85 cases of abortion in a 9-month period. This would mean that 17% (85/500) of the adult women, and perhaps even more, had an abortion in that year. Flavier (1980) in a study in rural communities of Cavite, finds that 17% of women of reproductive age say that they have had one or more induced abortions. In nearly half of these abortions, pharmaceutical tablets are used. He states that such tablets are the cheapest method for an abortion, in comparison with herbs, abdominal massage, and the 'catheter' method (inserting a thin catheter into the uterus, and waiting until bleeding commences).

During my own field work in urban slums of Manila I found that the pharmaceuticals most often used were high-dose hormonal products, which were sold under the brandnames *Gestex* and *Cumorit*. These high-dose oestrogen-progestin pills were on the market for the treatment of secondary amenorrhoea (absence of menstruation) of unknown origin. Formerly, they had been indicated and prescribed as pregnancy tests. The test worked as follows: if menstruation followed after use of the high dose of hormones, the woman was not pregnant. If menstruation did not occur, the woman was considered pregnant. The use of these products as a pregnancy test was stopped because of the possible effects of the hormones on the fetus. However, my study showed that most women, following the prescription of these medicines as pregnancy tests and the subsequent menstruation, had started to use the methods to induce a menstruation when their menstruation was delayed and they feared pregnancy (Hardon 1991). In the view of my respondents, the methods only worked when the fetus had not formed yet (within 2 months after a missed menstruation). The tablets then caused the 'blood clot' to come out. The efficacy was labelled as *pamparegla* (to induce a menstruation).

The life-story of Lina illustrates the way in which women resort to various forms of menstrual regulation and abortion:

Lina welcomed her first pregnancy after she had waited for 3 years. She gave birth normally, but 4 months after delivery she realized that she was again conceiving. She did not want a baby so soon, with a husband who turned out to be an alcoholic and who showed more concern for his *barkada* than his family. Panic sent her to several traditional midwives or *hilots* who squeezed and massaged the area below her navel as a method of abortion. The fetus was tough (*matibay*) as she had to go to 13 hilots but without any results. She stopped only when her insides felt swollen and inflamed and when she began to experience difficulty in breathing. The fetus survived and in January 1980 Lina gave birth at the local health center.

Afraid of having another pregnancy too soon, Lina tried taking *Noriday*, a progestogen oral pill (POP) which the centre had prescribed to her neighbour shortly after delivery. However, this was discontinued after two months as she said that she was not *hiyang* to it. She lost her appetite and subsequently her weight.

She often missed her periods after this, the earliest of which was only 6 months after her second delivery. She could not recall exactly how many times it happened. Though she never underwent pregnancy tests, she was sure she was pregnant as she felt her breasts become heavy and experienced morning sickness. To abort the pregnancy, she took different drugs. Again upon her neighbour's advice, she bought Cumorit, Gestex, quinine and a host of other drugs, the names of which she could not even recall, from the local pharmacy.

This became her practice until 1982 when she decided to proceed with her pregnancy as by that time her last child was already two years old. For her, 2 years was enough space between pregnancies, and she had wanted six children. She thus delivered her third baby in January 1983.

After childbirth, Lina again started to worry about conceiving too soon and thus in one of her well-baby visits to the centre, she accepted their recommendation for her husband to use condoms. Initially, the supply was provided by the centre for free. But later they just bought from a nearby commercial drugstore. She could not go back to the health centre burdened with having to take care of an infant, a toddler and a pre-schooler. But this was only for 3 months as her husband then refused to continue using the condoms, and no other method was substituted.

Thus, by September of that same year, Lina had already missed three periods. She asked around for a traditional midwife in the area. She found one who promised her that if Lina could only pay Pesos 200 (10 USD), she would be bleeding before she even reached the bottom of the steps of the *hilot's* home. The massage of the area below her navel was vigorous (*nilamas-lamas at piniga*), and the pain excruciating. But when Lina stood up, blood started to flow. She did not feel any fear then, she said, as she desperately wanted to stop the pregnancy.

Lina had been bleeding, not profusely though, for a month when she noticed that the blood coming out had turned to black with a foul odour. Initially, she did not pay any attention to this, thinking that the abortion was already complete. However, one night, after an exhausting day of scrubbing floors and doing the laundry at a nearby creek, she started to experience labour pains. Bleeding became profuse, and it was only after a chunk of flesh flowed out with the blood that she realized that the fetus had only then been aborted. It was at this point that Lina felt fear creep in at the thought that she could actually die of blood loss. The bleeding continued for around ten minutes until the placenta was finally expelled.

There was only her sister-in-law who assisted her, and at no point was she brought to the local health centre or a hospital as life then was hard, and she knew the health centres would not accept any cases of abortion.

Lina survived, but there was no time for her to rest. She had to recover while doing her regular routine of household chores.

Lina attributed her surviving the abortions to God's pity on her and her children.

The reproductive life-history of Lina moves from unwanted pregnancy to wanted one, with intermittent uses of contraceptives. The contraceptive pill was not *hiyang* for her. She lost her appetite and became thin. Her husband initially wanted to use condoms but then turned against them. Lina does want to regulate her fertility and resorts to all kinds of abortion practices, including high-dose hormonal drugs, which are available over the counter in pharmacies.

The research findings presented above give a dynamic view of fertility regulation in the Philippines. They situate contraception in women's life and relate contraceptive use to their socioeconomic living conditions. The findings reveal how women often feel uncomfortable about taking the Pill. It makes them weak and thin, can cause a 'hot head' and *kanser*. When their menstruation is delayed and they fear pregnancy, they often try to induce menstruation by means of high-dose hormonal products, other pharmaceutical products, or herbs. These interventions are not perceived to be hazardous to women's health. In fact, given the positive health effects attributed to menstruation, inducing a menstruation is valued positively, in a situation where the 'pregnancy' is perceived to only consist of a blood clot, and the fetus is not yet formed. Only when pills and herbs do not work, do women turn to the more dangerous methods such as massage and the so-called catheter method. This last method is the most risky option. The extent to which these methods work depends, according to the women, on how strong the fetus is attached to the womb, and how tough the fetus is. Abortion is not valued positively, but when resorted to because of economic hardship, people believe that God will understand.

A reason for people's lack of use of preventive methods is that these methods do not fit in the way they are forced to live their lives. Food for the day tends to be the priority concern. Problems are dealt with on a day-by-day basis. Thus, delays in menstruation and possible pregnancies are only dealt with when they are perceived to be problems, i.e. when the family simply cannot cope with another mouth to feed or has no way of caring for the child-to-be. Though not explicitly mentioned as a reason for non-use of the Pill, people seem to resist using preventive methods because *planning* not to have children does not make sense. Children are viewed as 'gifts of God'. This notion is reinforced by the Catholic Church, which also vehemently opposes the use of modern contraceptives, e.g. by pointing to the hazardous side-effects of these methods, such as *kanser*. The opposition of the church to contraception creates an environment in which people feel ambivalent towards its use. Even the family planning workers express such an ambivalence. A 1990 evaluation of their interactions with clients revealed that they emphasize the side-effects of the contraceptive pill, apparently in an attempt to prevent any claims afterwards from their clients concerning the effects of the methods on their health (ESCAP 1990).

Infertility regulation in Mozambique

Let us now turn to the second sociocultural setting, Montpuez in Mozambique, where Gerrits (1997) conducted fieldwork to describe the knowledge, perceptions and practices of infertile women concerning the causes of infertility, and the strategies they apply to find a solution for their problem. The women involved in the study all belonged to the ethnic group Macua. Most of them were Muslim, the dominant religion in the area. Almost half had never attended school. Most of them were small farmers.

Gerrits found that infertility is perceived to be a huge problem among these Macua women. The way in which Macua women cope with their infertility is very much related to the fact that the Macua have a matrilineal kinship system, i.e. descent is traced through the mother's line. Having children is very important in Macua culture, not only for the parents, but also for the members of the matrilineage, because children guarantee its continued existence. Childlessness is a problem that needs to be prevented. During initiation rites and pregnancy ceremonies, women and men are taught how they can have healthy offspring.

The government health services in town have only a few means to deal with the problem. They do a general gynaecological examination, ask about the reproductive history of the couple, test for STDs, do sperm analysis and consider the husband's occupational activities. Ways of treating infertility are even scarcer. STDs are treated with antibiotics, and the women are taught how to record their temperature in order to determine when ovulation occurs.

Only half of the 34 women who faced an infertility problem and were interviewed by Gerrits had used modern health care. Most of the times they could describe the examinations that they had had, but they did not understand the results. The women complained that prescribed medicines were often not available in the hospital pharmacy.

The Macua women were more satisfied with the herbal and spiritual treatments offered by traditional healers. The healers use explanations for infertility that the women are familiar with. Traditionally, infertility is related to problems with blood, gonorrhoea, or possession by spirits and witchcraft. In the case of problems with blood, it is said that the blood of the husband does not combine well with the blood of the woman. Sometimes, it is explicitly stated that the man's blood is too hot and poisonous. Gonorrhoea is thought to cause infertility by destroying the uterus.

The care provided by the healers is valued positively, because they speak the local language, have more time for the patients and allow the relatives to join in the consultation.

Apart from visiting traditional healers, the women also described seeking extramarital affairs, or a new husband, and they fostered children of relatives. Most of the interviewed infertile women reported having regular sexual relations with various partners, irrespective of being married or not. Some women said that the traditional healer had advised them to have an extramarital affair, to check if the blood of the other man was more compatible. If a woman becomes pregnant by another man than her husband, they say that they would not tell their husband. In case the husband ever finds out, they say that they would not be afraid of the consequences, even if it would lead to a divorce. The main goal was to have a child, not to remain with the husband.

When asked to compare their situation with that of fertile women, all women expressed feelings of sadness and jealousy. Some women expressed fear that their family would die out. Childless women mentioned the problem of lack of support from their children, now and in the future. Who will feed her and give her new clothes? Women who have never had children nor been pregnant cannot, for example, take part in the ceremonies organized for pregnant girls, *the nthaára*.

Women's experiences with infertility differ. Some women never become pregnant. Others do become pregnant, but suffer from miscarriages. Others have one or more children, but suffer from secondary infertility. Women can be infertile with one husband, and not with another. All women who find themselves not conceiving when desired seek treatments for the perceived condition of infertility. Some are cured, others continue to seek treatment, and again others finally decide to foster children.

Because of these different infertility trajectories, it is best not to conceptualize infertility as a static and unitary condition. The dynamic condition of infertility is well illustrated by the case of Genoveva:

> Genoveva is a 34-year-old woman, living in Montepuez, a district capital in the north of Mozambique. She belongs to the Macua. She married her first husband at a very young age, before she went through the initiation rites held after a girl has her first menstruation. Immediately after her marriage Genoveva became pregnant, but unfortunately this pregnancy ended in miscarriage. Then she decided to divorce, because she suspected that the blood of her husband did not combine with hers. She married

again and had one child with her second husband. She left him, because the man had slept with a daughter of her sister. Then she married again. The child stayed with Genoveva. While living with her third husband, she was not able to become pregnant. She visited several traditional healers and the medical doctor in the hospital in the hope of finding a solution for her infertility. According to the traditional healers, she became infertile because of incorrect handling of the umbilical cord after her first delivery. She did not record any result regarding the hospital diagnosis. She only knew that they gave her pills. After 13 years of marriage to her third husband, he decided to return to his place of birth, Magide. Genoveva wanted to accompany him, but her family did not allow her to do so. One year before the interview, she married again. Her fourth husband is with his other wife. Genoveva complains that her husband pays much more attention to his other wife than to her. He always stays only a few days with her. Therefore, she wants to divorce him. She has already asked permission of her relatives to do so.

The story of Genoveva illustrates the various causes attributed to infertility in Macua culture and the diverse therapeutic options that women have. We find that Genoveva divorces her husband because his blood does not combine with hers. She seeks help from traditional healers and from medical doctors. The case also shows the various ways in which women cope with the problem of infertility. The matrilineage influences the choices of women. Genoveva has to consult her relatives before divorcing her fourth husband. Her third husband has come to live with her. Genoveva wanted to follow him to his home region, but her family did not allow her to do so.

Towards context-specific reproductive health interventions

The assumption embedded in the objectives of the GRHPP project, within which the Mozambique and Philippines studies were conducted, is that understanding of the sociocultural dimensions of fertility regulation could lead to more culture- and gender-sensitive reproductive health programmes. The researchers aim to describe the needs and experiences of the target population as a prerequisite for such recommendations. Therefore, what can we recommend?

In Manila, from a reproductive health perspective, one would need to address the way in which women apply menstrual regulation, the extent to which they resort to unsafe abortions, and deal with the reasons of why women do not use contraceptives to control their fertility. The research in Manila reveals that women have their own views of the efficacy and safety of the contraceptive pill, which are influenced by the opposition of the Catholic Church towards contraception and the ambivalent attitude of grassroots family planning workers towards the contraceptive pill. Few women use modern methods of contraception, despite the fact that many do not want to become pregnant. The Pill is the most accessible and most used method, but it is often discontinued because of perceived side-effects. Menstrual regulation with herbs and pills is the first option chosen when a woman's menstruation is delayed, and when they fear they are pregnant without wanting to be. It is not perceived to be very dangerous. When women take these herbs or pills, menstruation can occur, probably because the woman was not pregnant in the first place. Only when the pills and herbs do not work do women turn to the more dangerous methods such as massage and the so-called catheter method. This last method is the most risky option.

It is important for health workers to engage in a dialogue with women on the safety and efficacy of existing fertility regulation practices. Biomedical information on the safety risks of the various abortion practices can be discussed with the women in health education sessions, and other options for fertility regulation than the Pill can be presented. Women to whom the Pill is not *hiyang* may feel more comfortable using the male condom or female-controlled barrier methods which have no systemic effects. Examples of female-controlled methods are the female condom and the diaphragm. These methods do not require the cooperation of men, who are sometimes reluctant to use condoms. Barrier methods have as an added advantage that they protect women against STDs. Women may also prefer a once-a-month hormonal injectable over the daily use of the contraceptive pill. The advantage of these injectables is that they do not need to be taken daily, while still resulting in a monthly bleeding which gives women the evidence that they are not pregnant. Women would also benefit from access to emergency contraception. They need to know that they can use ordinary contraceptive pills within 72 h after the act to prevent pregnancy. Ideally, safe menstrual regulation should be available to women who think they are pregnant and do not want to be. In Bangladesh, women can get such services, which consists of a dilation and curettage procedure, within 49 days after the missed menstrual period. No pregnancy test is done, and therefore the procedure legally does not classify as an abortion, which is illegal in Bangladesh, as it is in the Philippines (Hardon & Hayes 1997). Early intervention is congruent in the Philippines with women's notions that before 2 months there is only a blood clot, not yet a fetus.

Formulating such gender- and culture-sensitive interventions to address the problem of infertility in Mozambique is more difficult. The main problem is that biomedical treatments of infertility are generally inaccessible to people who live in poor countries. New reproductive technologies such as in vitro fertilization (IVF) tend to be restricted to the rich who can visit expensive private medical centres in the capitals of developing countries. What then can we recommend to a reproductive health programme that wants to deal with the problem of infertility in Mozambique? First of all, the health workers would need to respect the notions of infertility that people have, the traditional therapies that they use, and the ways in which they cope with the problem. The role that biomedicine can play in the Mozambique context is relatively limited. What health workers can do is reinforce the notion among the Macua that infertility is related to STDs. They can advocate the use of condoms to prevent the transmission of such diseases and related infertility. Also, when STDs occur, the services can ensure appropriate diagnosis and treatment. Apart from these preventive measures, there is a need to improve the patient-health worker communication during infertility consults. The study has shown that infertile women have little understanding of the diagnostic procedures and the therapies provided at the health services. Awareness of cultural notions of infertility can contribute to improved communication. In addition, an assessment is needed of the ways in which diagnostic facilities and curative services can be strengthened. Given the impossibility of introducing complex technologies such as IVF at the district level of health care, one can seek those treatments that are relatively cost-effective, for example donor insemination, stimulating coitus at the moment of ovulation, better means of ovulation monitoring, and treatment of hormonal disturbances. Some of the infertile couples could benefit from these therapeutic options, as well as from the improved prevention and treatment of STDs.

Reflections on the implementation of reproductive health care

The above case studies suggest that broadening family planning programmes to include other components of reproductive health care, such as the prevention and treatment of infertility and STDs, and safe menstrual regulation is important. Fertility regulation is in women's views integrally linked with health and disease. According to them, a lack of menstrual flow can cause ill health and even cancer. STDs are related to infertility. Comprehensive care is needed that considers the relations between family planning, abortion, infertility, STDs and general feelings of well-being and health.

Because of the weak operationalization of the reproductive health care approach, policy-makers and programme-managers in developing countries find it difficult to implement the revolutionary changes in the provision and implementation of family planning and health care required. First of all, they will need to review the services that are currently being offered and reflect on those that are missing. The extent to which family planning is integrated with other health care services at the district and community levels needs to be assessed. In some countries family planning is still a vertical programme, in other countries the programme is integrated in the mother and child care (MCH) component of primary health care. Reproductive health care policies need to be developed that specify at the national level what the aims of the policy are, and how the policy is to be implemented.

At the district level of health care, district health teams and PHC programme managers need to implement the reproductive health care policies, considering the specific problems that occur in the regions. Specific reproductive health interventions need to be defined in consultation with the people who are supposed to benefit from them. Such care needs to be context-specific and need-oriented. It does not make sense to broaden PHC services to include various new components of reproductive health care based on cost-effectiveness analysis, without first consulting the people concerned. We can learn from the Philippine family planning programme that care which does not consider people's views and practices is not efficient.

Health workers at the local level should play a key role in contextualizing reproductive health care. They work at the interface of national planning priorities and locally felt problems and needs. As Streefland (1994: 217) has argued: 'service organizations can become learning organizations which are able to provide their products effectively and with continuity. For this they need specific sets of instruments to acquire the information necessary for their learning. They also need training and reorientation to enable their staff to use the instruments effectively, including the preparation and the pretesting of tools and collection and analysis of data.' Staff time, technical support and resources need to be provided to enable such learning processes. The partner of the GRHPP in the Philippines, Health Action Information Network (HAIN), has set up a useful model for such training in the Philippines. Based on ethnographic research on young people's sexuality and AIDS, HAIN is now involved in a series of workshops and training sessions for local level health staff in Philippine municipalities. The health workers are informed about the HIV/AIDS risks and other health problems that young people are confronted with. They are then provided with seed grants with which they can do a study in their own service areas on the ways in which people deal locally with sexuality and protect themselves against STDs and HIV. The data are discussed in a follow-up session, during which context-specific reproductive health interventions are defined. Implementation of these interventions falls under the authority of these local level health workers.

Last but not least: involving men!

Finally, a word about the involvement of men. A challenge to all actors involved in the process of formulating and implementing reproductive health care is finding ways to involve men. Too often, men are defined as the problem: not wanting to use condoms to protect their partners from STDs, abandoning their wives when they are infertile, not caring about the consequences of unprotected sex. Consequently, women are seen to be victims. Involving men in the formulation of reproductive health programmes will enhance their involvement in the reproductive health care efforts and lead to new ideas about men's health and reproductive rights and responsibilities. It is therefore essential that local level learning processes include men in defining problems and needs.

Notes

1 I am indebted to my colleague Trudie Gerrits who generously shared her research results on infertility in Mozambique. Michael Tan, and Ruth van Zorge shared their data on fertility regulation in Manila.
2 The GRHPP project is coordinated by the Medical Anthropology Unit of the University of Amsterdam and Health Action Information Network in the Philippines and El Collegio del Sur (ECOSUR) in Mexico.

3 The research projects conducted in these countries have in common that they are conducted among relatively marginal populations: urban and rural poor, immigrants, and minorities.

4 The data that I present have been collected in urban poor settings in Manila, where I did fieldwork originally in 1987 (Hardon 1991) and have returned regularly since, and where researchers of the GRHPP partner agency in the Philippines, Health Action Information Network (HAIN), are conducting studies, and where a Masters student of mine, Ruth van Zorge, has recently conducted research. The data have not been thoroughly analyzed yet, but serve to illustrate the types of findings that are emerging from the ongoing GRHPP projects.

Literature

Aitken, I. & L. Reichenbach
    1994   'Reproductive and sexual health services: expanding access and enhancing quality.' In: I.G. Sen, A. Germain & L.C. Chen (eds), *Population Policies reconsidered: health, empowerment and rights*. Harvard Series on Population and International Health. Boston: Harvard University Press, pp. 177-193.

Alcala, M.
    1994   *Action for the 21st century. Reproductive health and rights for all.* Summary report of recommended actions of reproductive health and rights in the Cairo ICPD Program of Action. New York: Family Care International.

ESCAP
    1990   *Knowledge and attitudes of grassroots family planning workers about contraceptive methods, the Philippines.* Population Studies Series 86G. Bangkok: ESCAP.

Flavier J.M. & C.H.C. Chen
    1980   'Induced abortion in rural villages of Cavite, the Philippines: Knowledge, attitudes and practice.' *Studies in Family Planning* 2(2): 65-71.

Germain, A. & J. Ordway
    1989   *Population control and women's health: Balancing the scales.* New York: International Women's Health Coalition.

Gerrits, T.
    1997   'Social and cultural aspects of infertility in Mozambique.' *Patient Education and Counseling* 31: 39-48.

Greenhalgh, S (ed.)
    1995   *Situating fertility: anthropology and demographic inquiry.* Cambridge: Cambridge University Press.

Inhorn, M.C.
1994   'Ethnography, epidemiology and infertility in Egypt.' *Social Science and Medicine* 39(5): 671-86.

Jocano, L.F.
1975   *Slum as a way of life. A study of coping behavior in an urban environment.* Quezon-city: New day publishers.

Hardon, A.P.
1991   *Confronting ill-health: self-care, medicines and the poor in Manila.* Quezon-city: HAIN.
1992   'That drug is hiyang for me: lay perceptions of the efficacy of drugs in Manila, Philippines.' *Central Issues in Anthropology* 10: 86-93.

Jain, A.K.
1992   *Managing quality of care in population programs.* Hartford: Kumarian Press.

NDS
1993   *National Demographic Survey, the Philippines.* National Statistics Office. Calverton MA: Macro International Inc.

Streefland, P.
1994   'Enhancing the flexibility of service organizations: An effective contribution to sustainable development.' In: Liber Amicorum E.W. Hommes. M.M. Skutsch, H.M. Opdam & N.G. Schulte Nordhold (eds), *Towards sustainable development.* Enschede: Technology and Development Group, University of Twente, pp. 203-228.

Tan, M.L
1997   *Magaling ng Gamot.* PHD thesis, University of Amsterdam.

WHO/UNICEF
1978   *The declaration of Alma Ata.* Geneva: WHO.

WHO
1987   'Infections, pregnancies and infertility: Perspectives on prevention.' *Fertility and Sterility* 47: 964-968.
1997   'The global burden of reproductive ill-health.' *Progress in Human Reproduction Research* 42: 2-3.

World Bank
1993   *The World Development Report 1993: Investing in Health.* New York: OUP.

CHAPTER VII

How to Improve Quality of Care in Africa:
Are Health Reforms the Beginning of an Answer?[1]

JARL CHABOT

In February 1997 I visited Guinee Bissau, a country that I have known since 1978 and have been involved with regularly ever since. With slightly more than 1 million inhabitants, it is a small country isolated from the rest of the world due to its lusophonia. It is also one of the poorest countries in Africa.

In 1978 I came to the country as a 'suppletion expert', working in a line function for the government to set up a community health programme together with some 20 pioneer nurses and social workers in the southern province of Tombali. My boss was a Guinean nurse in charge of this new programme, an exceptional person, from whom I learned how to speak and relate to the people.

In 1997 I returned as part of a team of a large World Bank programme that supports the country technically and financially in the formulation and implementation of the National Health Development Programme (PNDS). My boss is the WB country officer, who tells me what to do and when to submit the pretty complex final report. Now a Pajero jeep comes to fetch me from the airport, and my boss insists that I stay in the cold and chilly Hotti Hotel at USD 100 a night, while before I slept with friends in the capital and showed disdain for those who went to sleep in the only reasonable hotel in town. It is clear that I have changed substantially.

But also the country has changed since the early days. Before, very little was available in the shops and at the markets, now almost everything is on hand for those who have the money to buy. Then, I had to order tyres for the bicycles of the nurses in Senegal in order to enable them to peddle to the villages, now all sorts of spare parts can be bought locally and assembled. Before we had to get even our beer through a formal request with signatures from officials, now all sorts of beer (mostly canned from Europe) can be bought in the smallest bars and clubs throughout the country.

In short, then we shared poverty, there was little equipment and few materials to develop the country, and even with money you could buy very little. Now we can develop the country as everything is available, but very few have the necessary money. Material conditions for development now seem better, but little development in the true sense of the word takes place. In fact, this is nothing new: the poor get (relatively) poorer and the rich become slowly more powerful and thus richer. No 'trickle down' is visible. On the contrary, people are more visibly exploited, and it appears difficult for them to organise themselves and demand that their needs be taken into account.

Professionally, I feel torn between improved planning with the involvement of a few people or more widespread and intensive participation but little progress. In fact, as a consultant I advise and suggest, but I do not become involved in the actual implementation, which is left to those who remain behind when I leave. Sometimes this gap between advice and execution is frustrating. Still, I feel fortunate to be able to come back regularly and discuss with those involved what has happened.

When people ask me whether I see progress in the country, I respond with 'I do not know'. For some yes, for many ...? When people ask me whether all that money brings positive change, I respond that indicators like infant mortality and death and birth rates seem to be improving, but slowly, painstakingly slowly.

With this personal introduction I want to highlight that not only the theory and practice of health care delivery have changed, but also that we, as long-term participants in health development, have changed, being moulded and transformed in the process. I shall now discuss some elements of the process of change in two countries, Guinee Bissau and Zambia. I have visited both countries recently, Guinee Bissau in January 1997 (World Bank 1997) and Zambia as a member of a multidisciplinary evaluation team of the Zambian Health Reforms in September 1996 (Draft evaluation report Zambia 1996). I shall present Guinee Bissau as an example of a Sectoral Investment Programme (SIP), that tries to initiate health reform in a more technical way, steered by the public health technicians of the Ministry of Health MOH, but with little political interest and support from the various political parties in the country. In Zambia the reform implies a change in the structure and organisation of the MOH. The change has become incorporated in the political discussion of the government and in the agenda of the ruling party. It is presented as a vision for the future. As the Minister of Health Katele

Kalumba says: 'we want to provide Zambians with equity of access to cost-effective, quality health as close to the family as possible' (Kalumba 1996).[1]

After a description of changes in the health service delivery systems and of the most important elements of the health reforms and the SIPs, I will use the experiences in these two countries to highlight some critical issues. Potentially, the changes envisaged can have profound and long-lasting consequences for the health of the urban and rural populations. Although to my knowledge no data are as yet available to 'prove' that the health of the people is improving, theoretical considerations and experiences to date do provide arguments that the SIPs and the reforms can be beneficial for substantial parts of the population.

Changes in health service delivery

Health service delivery systems have changed considerably over the last 30 years. While in the 1950s and 1960s emphasis lay on isolated disease control programmes (malaria, yaws, TB and schistosomiasis), in the late 1960s and the 1970s the importance of the basic health services (BHS) and the important role of the hospitals within the health care pyramid were stressed. Referrals and mobile clinics were introduced but not seriously promoted. Public health pursued smallpox control and vaccination programmes. The 1970s showed a growing dissatisfaction with this medically dominated system. This lead in 1978 to the Alma Ata declaration that fundamentally reoriented our view on health toward a holistic vision, where both consumers and providers had to play their part if health was to improve at all. Comprehensive PHC was the buzzword, and selective programmes were to be integrated into the health service delivery system. Health care was to be demystified and not to remain exclusively in the hands of the medical profession. The population was asked to participate in decision-making at least at the village and health centre level. Community-based health care (CBHC) with participation became one of the cornerstones of health development.

However the 1980s saw a growing deficit in financing health service delivery, which had been free of charge in most countries up to that time. Structural Adjustment Programmes (SAP) necessary to revitalise the national economies while containing the state budget had devastating effects on the social sectors (Bijlmakers & Harnmeijer 1995). SAPs paved the way for the introduction of user fees and the importance of cost-effectiveness as an evaluative indicator. The Bamako Initiative and the conference on district health care in Harare in 1987 provided landmarks in the process of changing PHC.

The following ailments, amongst others, of the health system at the time led to the more profound reforms and SIPs we witness today (Box 1).

Box 1

Ailments of the health system in most countries:
- Project-based approach: fragmentation;
- Multiplicity of projects impossible to manage by MoH;
- Resource allocation dominated by various stakeholders;
- Each donor has its own programme or geographical area;
- Duplication of resources and activities: endless missions;
- Inadequate planning and management of health services;
- Institutional and administrative paralysis;
- No reinforcement of MoH: no prioritisation.

The World Bank's *Investing in Health* (World Bank 1993) gave new impetus to policy discussions by stating clearly that investing in health is necessary to promote development. This publication finally gave a much needed signal to politicians and Ministries of Health that health mattered, that investing in health was economically sound and worthwhile and that the so-called 'social sectors' were very important to assure sustainable development. *Better Health in Africa* (World Bank 1994) provided the necessary content, by defining basic requirements and tools for a sustainable health care delivery system (Box 2).

Box 2

Requirements for Better Health in Africa (BHA)
- The concept of a two-layered district health delivery system that provides cost-effective packages of care;
- Decentralisation of authority to the district level;
- So-called 'essential health inputs': essential drugs, human resource development and a well-defined maintenance policy (for cars and equipment);
- An effective public/private mix in which both systems play their part and assure equity and sustainability.

[Source: Dubbeldam et al. 1996.]

This last publication certainly helped to arrive at an internationally accepted set of concepts, that facilitated the discussion on issues such as district health care, participation, decentralisation, the role of hospitals. In the wake of *Better Health in Africa*, health reforms and sectoral investment programmes (SIPS) came on the international agenda.

Health Sector Reforms

Health sector reforms, as defined by Conn et al. (1996: 44), is a process of fundamental change in policy and institutional arrangements guided by government and designed to improve the functioning and performance of the health sector and ultimately the health status of the population. Health reforms is now the catchword for organisational and institutional changes by governments to health services both in the North and in the South. In fact, some of the most important reforms in the South at this moment (like in Zambia and Ghana) have partly been inspired by experiences with previous reforms in the UK and the Scandinavian countries (Saltman 1995). In its various forms, the reforms aim to introduce 'managerialism' in public services, i.e. market-oriented approaches to service provision. Reforms not only redefine policy objectives and strategies, they also aim to reform the MOH. No wonder that the objectives and processes of the reforms are all politically loaded and complex to analyse. The WHO has brought together a group of experienced senior technical staff with a common interest in health policy and health reforms in the *Forum on health sector reform*.

In addition to the requirements for Better Health in Africa as mentioned in Box 2, I want to mention the most important elements addressed in these sectoral reforms (Box 3, source: Green 1996).

At a more general policy level, it appears that the goals of the health reforms are to reconcile the irreconcilable. In fact, they try to arrive at a 'fit' between general and widespread access to health care (equity) of acceptable standard (quality), which is effective and affordable (efficiency) (Figure 1). The problem is that when costs for the government are reduced by increasing the contribution of the population (Bamako Initiative), equity and coverage suffer. On the other hand, when efficiency is improved through decentralisation and an increased sense of ownership, as was tried in Zambia, quality might be sacrificed. What seems needed is to address these issues in different combinations and at different levels. Improvement of management at the central level (efficiency) should go together with an increase of quality of care to the patient at the health centre. Similarly, improved accessibility should not diminish the quality and effectiveness of care. Finding creative and practical answers to this sort of contradiction is the secret of successful and sustainable reforms.

Box 3

Important elements of Health Sector Reforms:

- Separation of normative (policy development) and executive (service delivery) functions of the MoH;
- Reduction of state role: emphasis on private sector involvement and NGO's;
- Increase of the market approach in the management of the public sector;
- Decentralisation of authority of government health services;
- Diversification of resources both centrally and in the periphery;
- Emphasis on the integration of vertical programmes, as those on control of TB and AIDS and on reproductive health.

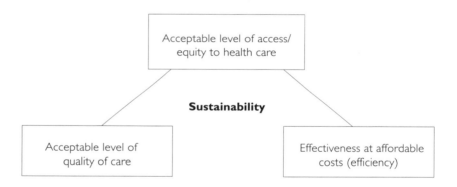

Figure 1   'Fit' of Health Sector Reform goals

Sectoral Investment Programmes

SIPS aim to improve the functioning and performance of the health delivery system. They function at a more technical level (Cassels & Janovsky 1996a; World Bank 1996). Nevertheless, the distinction between SIPS and health reforms is not always clear, as the redefinition of objectives and strategies of the health care delivery system itself might lead to changes in the organisational structure of the MOH. The important features of SIPS (summarised in

Box 4) reveal their significance as a tool for both the government and the donor community to improve health delivery.

Box 4

Characteristics of Sectoral Investment Programmes (SIP's):

- Sector wide in scope;
- Based on clear policy, strategy and priorities;
- Prepared by local stakeholders, with MoH in driving seat;
- Includes majority of donors active in the sector;
- Defines minimal package per level of care;
- Stresses common implementation and management arrangements;
- Budget is uniform, complete and transparent for all stakeholders;
- Minimises long-term technical assistance and mainly use of local technical assistance;
- Stops project-based work based on particular external preferences;
- Annual review of progress with MoH and all participating donors.

The elaboration of a SIP is a major exercise that took the MOH of Guinee Bissau more than 2 years to complete. It proved of tremendous value for the country to define its own strategy (including the definition of its minimal health care package and introduction of the *carte sanitaire* (health area) for effective coverage), its priorities (primary, secondary or tertiary care, the essential drugs programme, training programmes for human resource development) and the internal organisation needed to make its implementation feasible. In this way it not only resulted in a common framework, but also provided consensus and ownership in the MOH regarding what is needed in the years ahead.

At a different level, SIPs can contribute to a shift in power by strengthening the recipient countries' capability to direct and manage donor inputs. A prerequisite is that all donors channel their funds together with the government's own resources into a consolidated fund, called common pool or basket, without earmarking. This basket funding provides enormous potential for an MOH to re-establish their position in the driving seat and reinforce their sense of ownership in defining the health policies in their country. Finally, once the project-based approach is abandoned, fragmentation and duplication can be stopped, and common accounting and auditing systems elaborated. Subsequently, a system of transparent performance monitoring can be put in place. The potential for earning by a more efficient use of scarce resources is enormous, while the transparent budget, in which everybody can see what each stakeholder is contributing at what level and for what purpose, can create a sense of uniformity of purpose that is inspiring and rewarding for everybody involved. However, reality is seldom as bright as described here, and it often takes painstaking discussions and endless meetings to 'negotiate' acceptable formats for all donors involved. Much depends on the firmness and determination of the top civil servants within the MOH, on whether they succeed in getting all stakeholders to speak the same language and accept the same rules of the game.

Health reforms and SIP's: Examples from Zambia and Guinee Bissau

Organizational changes in Zambia

Zambia provides a fascinating example of the separation between the normative or policy-related functions of the MOH on the one hand and its operational tasks on the other (see Figure 2). At *the central level*, the MOH has been 'downsized' to a small body of about 100 civil servants responsible for political control, policy development, donor coordination, resource allocation, legislation and monitoring the performance of the operational organisation, the Central Board of Health (CBOH). This reduced MOH has delegated all responsibility for delivering health care within the country to the CBOH through a formal contract, that is reviewed annually (Koot 1997). The CBOH employs around 300-400 persons on a contract basis. Deliberately, no permanent contracts have been provided to the new staff of the CBOH, most of them being former civil servants from the MOH. This reorganisation strikingly attains two objectives in one move: it changes the staff composition in the health sector or even limits the number of civil servants, and it provides the opportunity to reselect the most capable staff for new and challenging tasks. At the same time, it also provides clarity of roles and tasks between MOH and CBOH.

The CBOH now functions as a sort of 'para-statal', and is still in the process of redefining its positions, salary scales, and internal lines of communications. Furthermore, the CBOH had to elaborate managerial guidelines, supervision schedules, financial reporting systems and annual contracts to the 58 District Health Boards (recently this number has been raised to 64 boards), that were created in most districts around two years ago, as well as in the so-called autonomous hospitals, that exist at the national and provincial level.

In the course of this major re-organisation process, it became apparent to the reformers that the *provincial level* provided an important obstacle for the reform. Prior to 1993, financial power was in the hands of the Provincial Permanent Secretary, but this added bureaucracy and paperwork without any major contribution to content and quality of the peripheral services. So, when the decentralisation was initiated and the districts received their money directly from the central level, much initiative and creativity became apparent at the district level, receiving technical support and supervision from the provincial level. But this support did not need to be linked with financial responsibility.

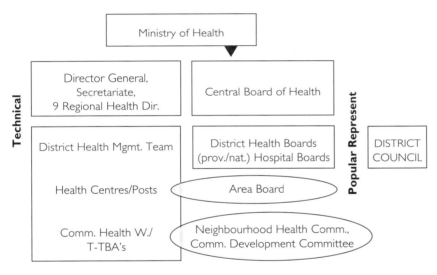

Figure 2 Organogram Health Sector Zambia

Recently, the MOH went even further: the provincial level now is no longer considered a separate layer within the health care pyramid. It is rather seen as the 'extended branch' of the CBOH. Its most important role is to strengthen district capacity, by supervising and monitoring the contract between CBOH and the District Health Boards. This second important feature of the Zambian reform is called 'delayering'. Again, a sweeping change has been made: a reduction of the CBOH bureaucracy and the number of civil servants it employs, and a complete review of the role and functions of the intermediate levels of the health care pyramid. Fewer layers of control imply more flexibility.

At the *district level* changes were initiated in 1993. All 58 district health management teams (DHMTs) from then on could manage budgets and handle money on the basis of approved annual plans. They received norms and guidelines explaining what these annual plans should look like, and 'waves of training seminars' were started all over the country. A specially created Health Reform Implementation Team (HRIT), together with the still operational provincial staff, supported the DHMTs in the elaboration of their district analysis, their definition of priorities and finally the elaboration of their budgets. It was also spelled out how much money in the budget could be spend by the DHMTs and on what sort of item (see Table 1). Once these annual district plans have been accepted, the money is send directly from the MOH, bypassing the provincial health structures. A strict 3-monthly financial reporting and disbursement schedule is in operation.

Table I Budget and Expenditure Ceilings, Zambia, 1996

Level	Minimum	Maximum
District Office	5 %	15 %
First Level Referral	20 %	40 %
Health Centre + Community	45 %	65 %

Note: Guidelines for the various bodies in the periphery have been prepared, that provide quite detailed instructions on how to plan and manage the services concerned. See for example the Handbook for district health board members (June 1996) and the District Health Plan guidelines for 1997 (version dated 27-06-1996).

With these important measures, the government of Zambia has shown its health personnel and its people that reforms can bring about change and improve morale. The newly available money in the periphery has created an outburst of activities: improvement of hospital wards, painting of hospitals, provision of blankets and also many seminars, meetings and discussions to inform staff about what was happening.

Recently, apart from the DHMTs that are operational in all districts, District Health Boards (DHBs) have been officially appointed by the Minister of Health (see Figure 2). They include representatives from communities within the district, private and NGO health providers (e.g. from missions), the local business community, the District Council (local government). The decentralisation of power to local government (District Councils) as a general policy of the Zambian government and the decentralisation first to the DHMTs and now to the DHBs initiated by the MOH raise many questions and provide interesting discussions. Presently, this process is still much debated, and the outcome is not yet clear. In particular the relation between MOH and the local government is not yet obvious. The DHBs have autonomy, for instance, in issues of financial management (e.g. regarding additional income generation and fee-setting) and in the important area of personnel policy. They can decide on vacancies, salaries, referrals within the district and new appointments. In this way the DHBs can hire and fire personnel. As the DHBs appear not yet well prepared for these new tasks, considerable anxiety exists amongst health staff at various levels. Many worry about whether their position, once it has been suppressed by the MOH, will automatically be re-opened by the DHBs. There is the possibility that all sorts of local influences and preferences will interfere.

The control of the DHBs over the District Health Management Team (DHMT) is the third major change implied in the Zambia reforms. Its outcome is difficult to predict at the moment. Whether the DHBs will be only a temporary measure is also not clear. The fact that its members have been partly appointed by the current Minister of Health and have received training in management seems to indicate that they could well become longer-lasting institutions with specific tasks to guide, supervise and control the health services in the district.

At *subdistrict level,* there are area boards supervising one or two health centres, and at *community level* Neighbourhood Health Committees have been created. In a few districts committees and boards are represented in the administrative body at the level above. The relation of Village Health Workers (VHWs) and Trained Birth Attendants with the Health Centre staff is still unclear. In some districts training of VHWs is still being planned, but in most no CBHC activities are currently taking place, nor is regular supervision of village level activities carried out.

The effect of the health reform in Zambia at these two most peripheral levels is still unclear: selection and installation of committees has taken place, but they are hardly operational. Money is often not trickling down to these committees, and the procedures for obtaining access to it are not always known at these levels. Frequency of supervision by the DHMT of the staff of the health centre (HC) level has improved, but in terms of quality much remains to be done. Momentum here seems to be faltering, and it remains to be seen whether the DHBs will show sufficient interest for the villages in their district to address this situation.

Equity in Zambia and Guinee Bissau

Both in Zambia and in Guinee Bissau the 'essential package of care' has been defined based on a standardised number of population (about 10,000 people) and reasonable estimates of coverage and attendance. This package of essential care at the HC level subsequently provides the basis for planning of infrastructure, personnel and drug requirements, including the definition of the expected output. Standardised treatment schedules, referral guides, equipment and maintenance schemes, health information systems still need to be worked out. The package also allows for a detailed definition of performance indicators, as has been proposed by the World Bank for Guinee Bissau (see Table 2). The Bank would like to use these indicators as the basis for the establishment of 'performance contracts' between the district authorities and the HC staff. It could motivate staff to reach the indicators established, if when doing so they will receive specific bonuses.

Table 2 Performance indicators for health centres

Criteria	10 points	5 points	0 points
Resources (max 20 points)			
General nurse + midwife or assistant	Yes	-	No
3 drugs + 2 vaccines available on % of 365 days	95	90-94	< 90
Process indicators (max 40 points)			
Outreach visits/month	4+2 - 3		< 2
Difference between expected vs. realized returns	< 5	5-10	> 10
Community participation (treasurer, president, 2 meetings)	Yes	-	No
% expected monthly visits	> 80	75-80	< 75
Results (max 40 points)			
% Delivery assistance	> 50	30-50	< 30
% 3 Antenatal visits	> 70	50-70	< 50
% 3 DPT-vaccinations	> 70	50-70	< 50
Curative consultations per person per year	> 0.35	0.2-0.35	< 0.20
Total score of performance	100	50	0

In Zambia, the reform has reduced the funding to the University Teaching Hospital from around 25% to 12% of the total health budget. This enabled the proportion of the budget for district spending in the country to increase from 45% to 57%. Nevertheless, distribution of personnel and money still follows the existing pattern of facilities, creating a bias in favour of areas that can provide adequate staff accommodation. However, not only personnel distribution is still far from ideal. In terms of gender distribution, very little has been improved. The composition of the CBOH, the DHB and the various other representative bodies does not guarantee at all an appropriate gender balance. Suggestions about including a certain percentage of women on the boards have been made, but are not always respected. Important decisions, including those regarding reproductive health initiatives, are taken without women being present. The interest of women as users and producers of health care are often not addressed specifically, not only in Zambia but also elsewhere (Standing 1997). This will have a detrimental effect on care for women and children under five.

Research into equity issues is important and could look more closely at the mechanisms of community participation and popular representation in the decentralised structures mentioned earlier. Attention for VHWS and TBAS is diminishing in most countries. In Guinee Bissau the national CBHC programme is seriously threatened, because the planning and management of the reforms consume all the available time of health staff. Representation of male and female villagers in HC and/or district committees is vital to assure that their interests are taken into account. However, to my knowledge very little research is done in this field. Social scientists together with public health staff should look urgently into this forgotten subject. Otherwise reforms will put an end to the importance of participation that was so forcefully promoted and adopted by all stakeholders in the PHC era.

User fees, cost-recovery and cost-sharing

In Zambia, user fees were introduced in 1993. Initially, no guidelines were provided and districts were left free to decide what the population had to pay. This created a lot of chaos. In 1994 regulations were given: a flat rate for each consultation, no charge for children under five and for the elderly, no charge for sufferers from chronic diseases nor for preventive services, as for instance vaccination. As a result, there was little consistency in the level of fees, the services for which charges were levied and the system granting exemptions. Although the main thrust of the Zambian reforms is about re-allocation of resources, in the minds of the public it is associated with user charges and no guarantee for availability of drugs at the health facility.

At the moment the situation is still not clear. Due to the drug-kit system, financed externally, drugs are available at the peripheral level, but very few drugs can be obtained at the (district) hospital level. Price setting for drugs and services by DHMT and/or DHB tends to increase prices for the public, as both look more at ways to make ends meet than at equity considerations. In an interview with the newly elected chairman of the District Health Board in Kapiri Mposhi, he expressed his conviction that fees in his district should go up 'to have more drugs, more beds and good equipment for the hospital'. He did not believe that part of the rural population would have problems to pay these higher fees: 'If you see what they spend on beer, I know they can spend the money on hospital fees'. Finally, he expressed his concern that the doctor of the DHMT should not do so much paperwork and workshops but rather take care of patients. 'If I were to run my business as they run their hospital, I would have been broke already a long time ago,' he added.

In conclusion, decentralisation to district level might lead to higher fees and thus to less equity and less attention for preventive work. Although this concern has been expressed earlier, it seems difficult to do something about it (Mills 1995). Therefore, representation of people from the area boards or from the neighbourhood health committees in the DHB will prove vital to make the voice of the population heard in these meetings.

In Guinee Bissau, the introduction of the Bamako Initiative has been on the agenda since 1993. However, apart from experiences in the Gabu district with specific support from UNICEF and an Italian NGO, no widespread cost-recovery has been introduced in practice, despite moral support from the MOH. The main reason for this is probably the tacit resistance from mainly vested interests of the medical profession and the pharmaceutical sector in the capital and some other urban areas. The decision to start the Bamako Initiative remained almost two years on the agenda of the Council of Ministers for no apparent reason. Only recently, through external donor pressure, was the uniform proposal of the MOH for the implementation of the Bamako Initiative at the national level endorsed. As the operational modalities are entirely decided by the technicians of the MOH, problems with consistency in the level of fees or with the diversity of district level decisions as in Zambia are not expected here.

Efficiency of health service delivery

Integration of so-called vertical programmes is an important component of health reforms. Its necessity is argued mainly for efficiency reasons. In Guinee Bissau the various vertical programmes have been merged into a disease control and a reproductive health programme. Whether AIDS will be part of disease control or reproductive health or remain a separate programme has not yet been decided. The need for integration becomes evident when we look at the refresher courses, seminars and workshops that the existing departments had planned. Once put together during the annual planning exercise, the plethora of courses for the district staff appeared so overwhelming that hardly any 'normal' days of work remained. All the days of the year were filled with courses for control of malaria, of TB, on rational use of essential drugs, training of trainers in community health, on reproductive health, as well as supervision and planning meetings. As these courses and meetings imply important opportunities to add money to the low salaries of the staff, widespread opposition can be expected against decisions to rationalise the training of health personnel in the various (vertical) programmes.

In Zambia, efficiency has been enhanced by concentrating the positions of all the heads of the vertical programmes in one person within the district health management team. He or she is responsible for the coordination and programming of all vertical programmes. Supervision of these programmes is a shared responsibility of all members of the team. However, the future roles and responsibilities of the former coordinators of vertical programmes are not yet clear. Their morale and commitment to the reforms appear rather low.

Coordination in the sense of more efficient use of transport and planning of supervisory visits has improved, but knowledge and experience have often not been integrated and shared with other staff. Support by 'vertical' staff at the central level to clinical staff in the OPD, hospital and HCs has been minimal. Technical advice, guidelines, treatment norms for malaria, safe motherhood, TB, HIV/AIDS and other fields are often not available in the peripheral consultation room. No practical suggestions on how districts could improve their interventions (like rapid and reliable diagnosis; reliable recording and reporting system) and how they should organise the training and supervision of their staff in these matters are available. In this way, the reforms risk leaving the vertical programmes floating, without proper direction and guidelines. This is a dangerous situation, as an important part of prevention and cure is being provided by these programmes.[3]

Zambia has concentrated its reforms on management issues like supervision, accountability and reporting. Although this is understandable, it seems that issues related to the direct provision of health care also need attention and should not be left out. Yet, the recent emphasis on issues related to quality of care, although still modest, is a hopeful sign of a more balanced reform process.

Human Resource Development

An important feature of the Zambian reforms is the transition of civil servants from jobs in the MOH to temporary contracts with the DHBs. The potential here is enormous: more flexibility in staff composition and financial allowances (salaries, improved working conditions), more emphasis on performance-related work assessment and, perhaps most important, the freedom for the MOH to introduce change and move away from the monolithic government structure that impedes any flexibility. However, there are also some important negative side-effects: reduction of job security often makes the best staff leave for the private sector, where they can make more money. Moreover, the possibility of abuse and personal favours, especially by the newly appointed district board members, is real, as few procedures exist to correct such a situation.

Unfortunately, during our visit it became apparent that few preparations had been made by the MOH for this enormous transition. District boards were not even clear themselves that they had been given the possibility to fire and recruit again (retrenchment) a substantial part of the MOH staff.

It further became clear during our visit in Zambia that human resource development (HRD) is perhaps the most critical and difficult element of the reform. However, it had been given the least attention (Martinez & Martineau 1996).

In Guinee Bissau, the SIP currently underway aims to provide one nurse and one midwife for each health zone of about 4000-8000 inhabitants. To create these 'multipurpose staff', housing for them will be built at all health facilities in the country, while career opportunities and other motivational incentives, like allowances, are being put into effect. In terms of manpower planning, the number of Guinean doctors in service and in training is considered sufficient for the future needs of the country.

Major training needs have been identified in the field of midwifery and nursing. As far as possible, auxiliary staff has already been upgraded to the level of general nurse/midwife. Another 150 midwives will be trained in the coming five years to fill the important gap of midwives in HCs around the country. Whether the MOH will be capable of actually sending these graduates to the rural areas remains to be seen. Furthermore, important investments will be provided for the upgrading of knowledge and skills of the existing medical staff.

Utilisation of health services

The mission to Zambia revealed that utilisation data over a longer time period provide imprecise information. National attendance rates appear to have gone down between 1991 and 1995 from 772 to 597/1000 population. Reasons for this decline include: introduction of user fees and changes in the fee structure in various districts; unavailability of drugs for longer periods; low quality of care (perceived and real); socio-economic problems like drought; the rise of the HIV-AIDS epidemic; and little attention to the specific needs of women. An analysis of the effects of the reforms on utilisation is, therefore, fraught with assumptions about the interference of other variables. Prospective long-term studies, both at the district and national levels are needed, combined with improvement in the registration of the many variables involved.

Health services are public goods, and the market model inherent in the reforms often does not clearly address the link between poverty and poor health: the least healthy often have the fewest resources to buy health care. Therefore, the effects of the reforms on the improvement of health of the urban and rural populations remains to be seen. Interdisciplinary research into these effects is needed.[4]

The comparison of utilization figures between Zambia and Guinee Bissau provides some striking differences. In Guinee Bissau, a nurse sees about 3-6 patients a day, while in Zambia this number is on average around 30-50 persons a day. A laboratory assistant performs about 1.5 blood tests a day in a Guinean health centre, while the Zambian colleague does about 10 times more tests a day. Average attendance figures in Guinee Bissau and Zambia show a tenfold difference: 0.1-0.3 NC/pp/yr (new consultation per person per year) versus 1-3 NC/pp/yr (for poor people this number drops to 0.05 pp/yr).

Reasons for these differences could be many: quality of care in Zambia seems better than in Guinee Bissau; people have more money to spend on health care; or coverage is more intense. It appears to me that in Guinee

Bissau people make more use of private care, including traditional healers, *marabouts* (faith healers), and vendors at the marketplace, whereas in Southern Africa, people probably use this private sector less frequently.

These differences are in my view representative not only for these two countries, but for substantial parts of Western and Southern Africa. Consequently, they may point towards different approaches to be used in the reforms. In Guinee Bissau and countries where utilization is equally low, measures to create demand should be emphasized, including different forms of education and information. In Zambia and similar situations, where demand is not a problem, emphasis should be put on improvement of patient flow, quality of care and standardisation.

Quality of care

During the Zambia evaluation, I saw nurses perform anamnesis, use weight charts, perform physical examinations, use decision trees and treatment protocols. Their attitude was better than observed normally in Western Africa, which might partly explain the important differences in utilisation rates. However, no standardised treatment protocols were available, and no use was made of the essential package of care, as originally defined by the reformers.

Gender sensitivity, like room for privacy and attendance of women by female nurses, was not observed. As Zambia is fortunate to have substantial numbers of female nurses (in contrast to Guinee Bissau, where all nurses are male and only midwives are female), it seems not too difficult to improve gender sensitivity during service delivery.

The overall lack of pharmaceuticals in hospitals and urban health centres mentioned earlier contributes greatly to the low level of perceived quality of care. As long as the drug supply to these institutions is not guaranteed, perceived quality is not likely to improve.

The MOH is aware that emphasis has been given predominantly to the management of health services, while less attention was paid to quality of care and the technical support of the vertical programmes. Recently specific attention has been focussed on these quality issues. Discussion is in process regarding whether contracting out of health care to private companies will improve the quality of care. According to Mills et al. (1997), contracting to the private-for-profit sector might reduce costs per patient, but does not enhance the quality of care in itself.

The donor community

Total per capita expenditure for health services from government revenues is USD 2 in Guinee Bissau and USD 8 in Zambia. In Zambia, about eight of the most important donors have agreed to contribute their funds to a basket that will be managed by the MOH. Districts receive each trimester a block grant to cover non-salary costs. No funds are earmarked for or controlled by specific vertical programmes. As earmarking of money by donors for specific programmes or districts has become impossible, it remains to be seen whether donors really will do this, when differences in opinion between donors and the MOH become apparent. The various administrative procedures that donors need to justify and check their expenses back home still need to be harmonised with the new set-up in a way acceptable for all stakeholders concerned.

In Guinee Bissau USD 8 is needed per capita each year, USD 6 of which is expected to come from the donor community. With substantial donor support and with improved coordination, this figure is likely to be achieved. Consequently, the funding of the National Health Development Programme for the coming five years has been assured. For the first time in the history of the country's health services, there exists a national budget per cost item (salaries, investment and recurrent costs), per district, per objective of the National Health Development Programme and per donor. At last, there is transparency, and that will help substantially to use the few available resources more efficiently.

Conclusion

Like primary health care, health reforms are almost by definition political in nature. Therefore, political leadership and public debate are a prerequisite for succesful reforms. SIPS appear more technical in content and approach. To become effective and operational, they should be linked with the political agenda of the reform. In this way their political implications will become explicit.

The current reforms provide the potential for improving health care delivery by trying to match efficiency, quality and equity. If donors and external agencies could harmonise their different agendas and if operational modalities are found to bring efficiency, quality and equity together into one coherent framework, substantial steps forward could result. However, as these elements often imply contradictory decisions, difficult choices have et be made. No shortcuts are available, and no easy answers can be given.

Cassels (1995: 48), the guru of health reforms, warns about too much optimism: 'Reform in the industrialised world has been designed to contend with sluggish economic growth, ageing populations, increasing expectations and rising costs ... but against a background of universal or near universal coverage and functioning institutions. In less developed countries reform strategies need to address the issues of extending coverage of basic services to under-served populations, improving poor service quality and addressing the inequitable distribution of resources in the context of very limited institutional capacity and funding'.

Notes

1 This paper was written in August 1997. In the following months informal news from Zambia indicated that major changes were about to happen due to court decisions in a dispute between the MOH and the Unions. These recent developments have not been included in this paper.

2 Cassels (1997) uses the concept Sector-Wide Approaches for Health Developments for both SIP's and Health Reforms.

3 Research on integration of the vertical programmes appears important. It should address questions like:
   – at what level should priorities be defined or strategies fixed?
   – at what level should fees be defined?
   – What are the effects of the reform on TB treatment and caseholding?
   – What does basket funding mean for the implementation of a vertical programme?
   – Can financial transparency be assured?
   – What is the District Health Board's perception of the importance of vertical programmes and of preventive activities like vaccination?

4 The WHO recently published an interesting agenda for research (Janovsky 1996) that could serve as a starting point for the development of a research programme in this field. Similarly, the EU published an overview of experiences with decentralisation in the health projects it funds (European Commission 1997).

Literature

Bijlmakers, L. & J.W. Harnmeijer
1995   'Discussions and conclusions.' In: J. Chabot, J.W. Harnmeijer &
       P.H. Streefland (eds), *African Primary Health Care in times of economic
       turbulence.* Amsterdam: KIT Press, pp. 119-149.

Cassels, A.
1995   'Health sector reform: Key issues in less developed countries.' *Journal of
       International Development* 7(3): 329-347.
1997   *A guide for sector-wide approaches for health development: concepts, issues
       and working arrangements.* WHO/ARA/97.12. Geneva: WHO.

Cassels, A. & K. Janovsky
1996a *Sectoral investment in health: Prescription or principles?* WHO Working
       paper. Geneva: WHO.
1996b *Reform of the health sector in Ghana and Zambia: Commonalities and
       contrasts.* WHO/SHS Current Concerns, paper no. 11. Geneva: WHO.

Chabot, J. & T. Sukwa
1996   *Summary report of the public health group on the Zambian Reform and
       the health system.* Joint comprehensive review of the Zambian health
       reform. n.pl.

Conn, C., Green, C. & J. Walley
1996   *Effective district health services in developing countries: A busy manager's
       guide to the literature.* An annotated bibliography. Development Biblio-
       graphy No. 13. IDS: Falmer.

Draft evaluation report
1996   *Joint comprehensive review of the Zambian Health Reforms.* Internal
       consensus report. n.pl.

Dubbeldam, R.P., H.T.J. Chabot & C.H. Varkevisser
1996   'Better Health in Africa: De nieuwe leidraad voor gezondheidszorg in
       Afrika?' *Medicus Tropicus* 34(4): 1-5.

European Commission
1997   *The decentralisation process in the health sector.* Health and development
       series, working paper No. 2. Brussels: EU.

Green, A.
1996   *How can managers of national leprosy programmes promote sustainability
       in the context of the changing composition and structure of the health sec-
       tor?* Paper for ILEP workshop, September 1996, Royal Tropical Institute,
       Amsterdam.

Janovsky, K.
1996   *Health policy and systems development, an agenda for research.* Geneva:
       WHO.

Kalumba, K.
 1996   *Towards an equity oriented policy of decentralisation in health systems under conditions of turbulance.* Internal working paper. Lusaka: MOH.

Koot, J.
 1997   'Decentralisation in the Health Reforms: the case of Zambia.' *Medicus Tropicus* 35(3): 2-4.

Kutzin, J.
 1994   *Experience with organizational and financing reform of the health sector.* WHO/SHS Current Concerns, paper no. 8. Geneva: WHO.

Martinez, J. & T. Martineau
 1996   *Proceedings of the workshop on human resources and health sector reforms, research and development priorities in developing countries.* International Health Division, Liverpool School of Tropical Medicine. Liverpool: LSTM.

Mills, A.
 1995   'What are the real answers?' In: J. Chabot, J.W. Harnmeijer & P.H. Streefland (eds), *African Primary Health Care in times of economic turbulance.* Amsterdam: KIT Press, pp. 43-51.

Mills, A., C. Hongoro & J. Broomberg
 1997   'Improving the efficiency of district hospitals: is contracting an option?' *Tropical Medicine and International Health* 2(2): 116-126.

Saltman, R.
 1995   *Applying planned market logic to developing countries' health systems: an initial exploration.* Forum on health sector reforms, discussion paper no. 4. National health systems and policies unit. Geneva: WHO.

Standing, H.
 1997   'Gender and equity in health sector reform programmes: A review.' *Health Policy and Planning* 12(1): 1-18.

World Bank
 1993   *World Development Report 1993. Investing in Health.* Washington: World Bank.
 1994   *Better Health in Africa.* Washington: World Bank.
 1996   *Sector Investment Programs in the Africa Region: a review of implementation experience.* Working paper no. 28. Washington: World Bank.
 1997   *Aide Mémoire de la mission conjointe (Banque mondiale, OMS, UNICEF, Pays Bas) de pré-évaluation de la préparation du programme national de développement de la Santé (PNDS) en Guinee Bissau.* n.pl.

CHAPTER VIII

From Bench to Bush: Problems of Vaccine Development and their Analysis

STUART BLUME

The perspective of this paper derives from many years sociological research on the development of new medical technologies. Until recently, my focus was exclusively on electronic devices developed for and principally used in the industrialized world (Blume 1992, 1995). Among the assumptions and findings of this work are the following.

Technologies are flexible. The shift from a preliminary idea or vision of something being possible involves a series of choices through which the technology takes shape. Assumptions, preferences – for example regarding how a technology will ultimately be used – get built in during the development process. There is nothing inevitable about this: it may reflect all kinds of social negotiations. That is why we sometimes speak of the social construction of a technology.

The development process typically involves collaboration between a group of clinicians – often from a specific medical speciality – and a firm. They have a shared interest in technological innovation, which is associated with enhanced status for the one and profit for the other. Until the 1970s no other group (neither government nor consumers/patients) had much influence. Everyone believed in letting the innovation process proceed under its own steam.

During the course of the last 100 years, industrialized societies have increasingly come to think of a healthier future in terms of medical science and technology. We believe in and want to believe in the possibilities of science-based new technology to cure all possible bodily afflictions.

The mass media play an important role in reinforcing this faith in medical technology and in stimulating enthusiasm for one remarkable breakthrough after another. This is particularly important where consumer groups who do not necessarily see themselves as sick have to learn to see the new technology as something for them. Contraceptive technologies are probably one example, technologies for handicapped people another.

In 1995, prompted by Pieter Streefland and Anita Hardon, I began to think about vaccine development. The challenge for me was to see in what ways an analysis developed in relation to one type of medical technology, and to the industrialised world, can be extended or needs to be changed when turned on a very different sort of health care technology. In the intervening time, and with the invaluable assistance of Ingrid Geesink, I have begun to work on vaccine development. This paper reports on work which Ingrid and I have carried out together. A number of the issues which arise have been set aside. We have not addressed the issues involved in the selling of high tech devices to the health care systems of the developing world, although I know that there are important problems there. The focus is on the problems of developing technologies specifically tailored to the preventive health care needs of poor countries. Why vaccines? Because there is a widespread assumption in the international public health community that

> Apart from the provision of clean water, vaccines have exerted a more profound influence on world health than any other public health measure (Moxon 1990).

> Vaccines are among the most affordable and effective health interventions available today (Mitchell et al. 1993).

The Expanded Program on Immunization (EPI), launched by the WHO in the mid-1970s, is the reference point for all subsequent discussion. Success in the eradication of smallpox (certified by international declaration at the end of 1979) served as a powerful symbol of what can be achieved. This was perhaps the most important implication of all, as Fenner and his colleagues conclude, in their mammoth account of the eradication programme:

> The achievement of smallpox eradication demonstrated the potential of WHO as an organization within which all countries, whatever their beliefs and politics, could cooperate successfully in the pursuit of a common global objective. It encourages the hope that other challenges might likewise be addressed ... an important impetus was provided for new initiatives in, for example, immunization, diarrhoeal disease control and the prevention of blindness (Fenner et al. 1988: 1366).

Not only did this declared success have major practical implications, it seems to have been no less a symbol of hope for scientists: hope that the eradication of other diseases would indeed be feasible. Fenner and his colleagues suggest that, for scientists, this very feasibility was the most important lesson to be learned from the programme. Perhaps the same might have been said of policy makers, for 'eradication', for example of polio, has since become an important goal for national and international public health policy makers. Nearly two decades later, and aware of the complexity of many viral diseases in particular, not all scientists are convinced of the wisdom of eradication strategies (Osterhaus 1997).

The account of the EPI, on which almost all authors seem to agree, is one of remarkable success in the face of considerable obstacles, increasingly tempered by concern at major problems standing in the way of further progress both in vaccination and in vaccine development.

In the course of the 1980s, international attention turned from satisfaction at what had already been achieved through the EPI to concern at what still had to be achieved. It was partly that many children remained to be reached, particularly in some of the remotest and poorest regions of the world. Economic analysis seemed to support the need to extend coverage. But there was also another sort of problem, which concerned the adequacy of the vaccines available. Was sufficient effort being devoted to improving the quality of the vaccines available within the EPI and, indeed, to developing suitable new ones? Didn't science have more to offer?

Commitment to vaccine development

The problem was becoming clear enough. Many of the vaccines currently in use are far from ideal under the circumstances pertaining in many developing countries. For example, since many vaccines are highly sensitive to temperature, their efficacy declining rapidly with rising temperature, they have to be maintained at low temperatures from the time of production to the time of use. This 'cold chain' is very difficult to maintain in many developing countries and contributes significantly to the costs of vaccination programmes. Failure here is frequently identified as a cause of the failure of vaccination programmes, and the relative stability of smallpox vaccine has indeed been put forwards as a reason for the success of that programme.[1] Enhanced heat stability is thus one vital aspect in terms of which, it is commonly argued, many existing vaccines – perhaps particularly oral polio vaccine – need to be improved.[2]

Is the problem one of the lack of scientific knowledge? Sometimes, of course, it is. Developing a vaccine against AIDS or malaria (or indeed any parasitic disease) poses very difficult scientific problems.[3] Fundamental knowledge is gradually being accumulated. However, as a recent survey of leading vaccine scientists, policy-makers and manufacturers showed, more is involved than lack of fundamental knowledge (Cohen 1994: 1371). This survey suggested that, in addition to scientific unknowns, 'the field lacks the strong leadership and funding to speed progress'.

A 1986 report from the Institute of Medicine of the US National Academy of Sciences produced a long list of pathogens against which vaccines were urgently needed in developing countries, all of which ought to be producible within a decade (IoM 1986). The list included vaccines against rotavirus and *Shigella, Plasmodium* (responsible for malaria), hepatitis B and the *Streptococci.*

Why were vaccines for which a clear health need existed and which scientifically speaking seemed within reach nevertheless not being developed? This question looms large in the public health perspective on 'the vaccine problem'. It is partly a matter of economics. Ten years ago the cost of developing a new vaccine was estimated at anything between USD 10 and 50 million (Mitchell et al. 1993). As you move from research to development, to large-scale clinical trials and then to setting up production facilities, costs rise rapidly.

> As a consequence, most vaccine development – especially the late stages –
> is sponsored by for-profit institutions in industrialized countries; these
> companies generally have not perceived the developing country market
> to be sufficiently lucrative as to justify development of vaccines primarily
> for that market (Hausdorff 1996).

Although there are important public sector institutions in the vaccine field (including RIVM in the Netherlands and the new International Vaccine Institute in South Korea) and although 70% of EPI vaccines used in developing countries are actually produced in those countries, the general view is that – at this moment – only the multinational pharmaceutical companies have the resources and the expertise necessary to develop new vaccines.[4] In the 1960s and 1970s one pharmaceutical company after another withdrew from the vaccine field. The lack of commitment of those companies, at least until recently, has been partly a matter of perceived costs and perceived benefits.

Whilst the size and profitability of the market may have been the most obvious factors discouraging major pharmaceutical firms from investing in vaccine development, they are not the only ones. Three others seem to be:

the problem of liability, (lack of) patent protection available in many developing countries, and the problems involved in setting up clinical trials. Petricciani and colleagues from the WHO suggest that liability – the fear of being wrong – may be a significant element in the thinking both of corporations and of regulatory agencies (Petricciani et al. 1989). What if a batch of vaccines were to contain active viruses, or give rise to unexpected side effects? Compensation claimed from the supplier could be vast. In the USA legislation has been passed limiting the liability of commercial vaccine producers, for fear that the country's supplies of vaccines would otherwise be at risk.

The problem of patenting, or intellectual property rights, is an extremely complex one because of widely differing governmental philosophies (Basch 1994: l29-36). The kind and duration of protection given by patent legislation differs greatly from country to country. In some countries it may be as little as five years; in others only processes and not products may be protected (so that patented products can be legally made by other processes); whilst in some countries commodities considered to be for 'the general good' of the people are simply not patentable. The issue may affect in particular a company's relations with the more advanced developing countries which themselves possess a scientific and technological infrastructure and competent local producers.

I shall consider the specific question of clinical trials in a little more detail presently. We need to focus now on some of the issues involved in the actual development of a new vaccine.

There is another issue which may be relevant in some cases but which we will not discuss. It relates to the fact that interest in developing a vaccine may be diminished when an effective therapy seems to be just around the corner. That has generally been the case in the field of malaria and may have occurred more recently with regard to leprosy.[5] In this context, Surabhi Tandon's study of leprosy vaccine development in India shows that many scientists committed to the development of therapeutic agents are critical of vaccine development work (Tandon 1996).

Some conceptual problems relating to vaccine development

It is perhaps worth returning briefly to the perspective underlying this paper. Technologies, for me, are developed through a constant process of choice: whether to go this way or that way; whether enough is known to justify taking the next step... At each point of choice or decision, the researchers, clinicians, industrialists involved have to assess what has been achieved to date. Does it seem to work? Is it safe enough? What I want to focus on is the way in which values, assumptions, social processes of negotiation play a role in vaccine development.

What do we mean by 'safety' and 'efficacy'?

In the course of developing a vaccine, moving from experiment to clinical trial, hypotheses relating to its safety and possible efficacy are endlessly made and revised. That a vaccine is accepted as 'safe' depends upon agreement regarding appropriate proofs of safety. That these proofs are far from self-evident can be seen from Millman's account of the development of hepatitis B vaccine. Safety was initially established on the basis of certain tests on chimpanzees. Going on to discuss the question of the high cost of the vaccine (this is a 1982 lecture: the price has subsequently fallen immensely), Millman writes:

> If the major contributing cost is safety testing, and we know that this is costly because it involves chimpanzee testing and a holding period of up to six months, then perhaps we should extend our efforts to finding alternative safety tests. This is not an impossible idea if one considers that there are now available [various DNA tests]. Can we determine whether these tests, on a product which is manufactured under the most rigid conditions... are sensitive enough? (Millman, 1984: 146).

In other words, reliance on particular tests of safety depends upon prior consensus regarding their adequacy/sensitivity being reached. We might go on to say that belief in the safety of a vaccine builds up (rather than being established definitively by any single test or series of tests). Still on hepatitis, McLean et al. (from Merck Research Lab) – now discussing a later stage in the process – discuss safety not by reference to Millman's chimpanzees, but to a criterion appropriate to clinical trials in humans. The vaccine is then deemed to be safe because of the lack of ('serious') adverse reactions in more than 19,000 volunteers followed for up to eight years in the course of the trial (McLean 1984). Safety, in other words, is a relative concept, defined by reference to subsequent steps to be taken: moving from animals to volunteers, volunteers to large trial populations, trial populations to routine programmes. At each step the question is posed: Can the next step justifiably be taken?

The issue of difficulties in the way of reaching agreement (not now about the nature of appropriate tests but regarding the interpretation of their outcomes) then arises. This is most obviously so where trials or other studies yield contradictory results. What you find – and that is fascinating for a sociologist of science – is a process through which contradictory results are nevertheless made to yield a coherent picture. A good example is provided by vaccination against tuberculosis with BCG (Eickhoff 1988). This is a complicated and interesting case both by virtue of differences in epidemiology of the disease between different regions and because of major differences in the local strains of BCG vaccine used in many countries.

Eickhoff draws attention to the unusual fact that no less than 8 large controlled trials of BCG have been carried out in humans (ranging from a US trial between 1935 and 1938 to an Indian trial between 1968 and 1971). Their results showed percentage protection ranging from 0% to 80%, so that no simple answer to the question of the vaccine's efficacy emerges. The author goes on to consider hypotheses which might explain these differences, and hence yield a more convincing and coherent picture. One possibility is that of methodological differences. A previous study had indeed come to the conclusion that the trials showing the highest efficacy were also those with the highest methodological and statistical rigour. Six other possible explanations of the failure of certain trials to yield positive results are then discussed (thus not of the fact that others yielded positive results). Particular attention is devoted to the last – Chingleput – trial, conducted in Southern India and which, it was hoped, would yield a definitive answer. The result, zero protection, was not what had been hoped for.

> The initial findings reported from the Chingleput trial represented more than simply an unpleasant surprise for public health officials throughout the world ... An unprecedented situation has evolved in which the effectiveness of a possibly very useful and, in fact, very widely administered tuberculosis contra measure has been seriously challenged...
>
> After the results [...] had been published and assessed, a WHO study group convened and recommended that the use of BCG vaccine on a worldwide basis should be continued, particularly in infants and children. In most developing countries, the current policy is to vaccinate newborns or very young infants. Although the very great need for additional information was pointed out, it was recommended that, in view of the safety of BCG vaccine and the lack of other effective means of tuberculosis control in developing countries, it would be prudent to continue using BCG vaccine for infants and children[6] (Eickhoff 1988: 383).

This case suggests a trade-off, in effect, between safety and efficacy. If there is no evidence that a vaccine is not safe, then the risk of using a potentially ineffective vaccine can more readily be accepted. It also suggests that decision-making may often be based on more than efficacy data alone. Here, the lack of any alternative is cited as a reason for continuing use of the vaccine.

How are data to be collected?

The controlled or randomized clinical trial is almost universally accepted as the most rational, the most scientific possible way of gathering data on a vaccine's efficacy. The conventional wisdom has it that initiation of a clinical trial is a rational consequence of accumulated knowledge based on laboratory experiments and animal models. At a certain moment available knowledge is sufficient to take this next step.

The practice isn't quite so 'objective'. In deciding whether (and, as I shall explain below, where) to initiate a clinical trial, more is entailed than the unambiguous interpretation of unequivocal data. Here are two examples showing the place of judgement and of values in deciding whether or not to conduct a large-scale trial. The first relates to the (Salk) polio vaccine, the second to an HIV vaccine.

In 1953 plans were laid to mount the largest clinical trial ever conducted, in order to assess the efficacy of Salk's recently discovered vaccine (Brandt 1978). Safety, it was stressed by those supporting the idea of clinical trials, had already been established ... though there were still major doubts as to whether manufacturers would be able to produce safe vaccine on the scale needed.[7] As the trials approached, 'scientific opposition remained formidable': various scientists were not convinced that the killed vaccine could be made safe enough, and a senior official of the US Public Health Service argued that the trials be postponed. However, as Brandt points out, 'the government had no legal means of postponing the trial' (which was financed by an independent body, the National Foundation for Infantile Paralysis). Not only that, but public expectations were enormous, built up by vast media coverage and by the National Foundation as part of the fund-raising by which it financed research and the trials.

In the case of recent trials of an HIV vaccine, scientific disagreement also emerged.[8] In late 1994 a WHO committee approved HIV vaccine testing in developing countries even though the (American) National Institutes of Health had decided not to go ahead with trials in the USA. Two members of the WHO committee have explained and justified the decision taken

(Moore & Anderson 1994). Whilst they recognize that some might attribute this decision to a differential morality regarding experimentation on the populations of developed and less developed countries, this is not the basis of their argument. Their basic argument hinges on the notion of risk. To establish a clinical trial implies that the likely benefits to the population are assumed to be greater than the possible dangers. Moore and Anderson argue that in respect to a population in which infection is largely restricted to high-risk groups (e.g. the USA), the justification is less than in a population such as in many developing countries ('where the prevalence of infection in pregnant women attending antenatal clinics in urban centres has reached 20% or more'). But even if committee members agreed with this basic assumption, their assessments of the likely efficacy of vaccines to be tested differed widely. Some took the view that the protection afforded to an individual would be so slight as to be insignificant on a population basis.

> This view tended to be held by researchers who had studied the immune response to subunit vaccines in human and animal models, whereas clinical scientists and epidemiologists were generally less swayed by uncertainties over which immunological markers best correlated with protection, or disagreement about the relevance of HIV-1 infections in chimpanzees ... Clinicians and epidemiologists argued that the only ways to determine efficacy is to run an efficacy trial (Moore & Anderson 1994).[9]

These kinds of differences in expert opinion, in so far as they become accessible, are an especially valuable resource in trying to show the socially constructed nature of knowledge and expertise.

It is important to look at ideas regarding how a trial population is to be selected. Two sorts of arguments are advanced here. Some argue for the importance of focusing on high-risk groups. This ensures that data which are the most unambiguous possible can be collected in a limited time. Knowledge of what the high-risk groups are then becomes important both for defining priorities for a vaccination programme and in deciding where to conduct a trial. Carrying out the trial in a population showing a high incidence ought to provide statistically meaningful results faster and more cheaply.

There may, however, be practical problems with finding an appropriate trial population, for example, in testing new vaccines against tuberculosis and leprosy. Because of the fact that BCG is widely used, it is difficult to find young populations anywhere in the world that are at any appreciable risk of tuberculosis yet have not been exposed to extensive BCG vaccination. Most of the high-risk populations that have not been exposed to BCG vaccination (like older individuals or the indigent in developed countries) are probably not suitable for the long-term follow-up required in vaccine trials. This scarcity of BCG-free populations means that careful long-range planning would be needed for future trials (Fine 1987: 357).

The competing perspective emphasizes the representativeness of the trial population in relation to that ultimately to be offered the vaccine. The notions of the acceptability and the accessibility of the trial to this population then arise. In his study of AIDS activists, Epstein explains their demand that clinical trial populations should be 'more fully representative of the different social groups affected by the epidemic' (Epstein 1995). They argued, in other words, that all affected groups in the population should have the *right of access* to trials of potentially beneficial new drugs. This right, rather than scientific convention, should govern the selection of trial populations. This obviously relates to one of the major discussion points in relation to clinical trials: the question of their ethics.

The principal issue which has emerged here is that of the acceptability of denying a possibly life-saving vaccine (or therapy) *believed safe and effective* (or else the trials would not be initiated) to a control group. The issue arose powerfully, and in practice, in the setting up of the first Salk polio vaccine trials. The original plan was to compare rates of polio among a group of vaccinated volunteers and non-vaccinated control children. The group overseeing the trial insisted on the need for 'double blinding', so that some volunteers would receive placebo. Salk was furious, arguing that if – as was likely – some of the volunteers contracted polio, he would feel personally responsible. Brandt writes:

> In a sense, Salk favoured an early limited distribution of the vaccine as a test for efficiency, not a carefully controlled, scientifically conducted examination. Sure of the safety and efficacy of his vaccine, he actually jeopardized its full acceptance in the medical community. (Brandt 1978).

The conduct of clinical trials is made far more complex when extended across national borders. Developed-country scientists working with Third World populations are often accused of 'cultural imperialis', especially when local people are consulted only marginally or not at all about the programme. Allegations of unethical conduct are made against those who give the appearance of selecting populations that are docile, uninformed, and unlikely to object to being used as test objects.

When populations are difficult to obtain in the researchers' own country, either because of the attitudes of the population or legal restraints on human experimentation, investigators may look to other countries where, for reasons of poverty, ignorance, or lack of legislative restraints, they can find populations available for experimentation. Manufacturers are very well aware of these problems. The dangers of being accused of unethical conduct, of 'abusing' a poor and ignorant population unprotected by adequate legislation, are widely recognized. International guidelines require investigators from one country working in another to apply ethical standards equivalent to those obtaining in their own country (Basch 1994: 89). It has been pointed out that the 'informed consent' required of a participant in a clinical trial is a concept which may translate only with difficulty into other cultures.[10]

I have been trying to weave together two rather different kinds of analysis relating to vaccine development. There is a well-established analysis of a roughly economic kind. The development of vaccines principally for poor countries is too risky and offers too little likelihood of profit to be of interest to multinational pharmaceutical companies. The less familiar analysis is sociological, and it concerns the process by which vaccines get developed or improved. It tries to disclose the values, assumptions and social processes through which vaccines (or any other technology) are endowed with specific features. The first analysis, in other words, addresses the problem of increasing investment in vaccine development and improvement, whilst the second relates to the social acceptability of the vaccines we get.

Of course, there are critics who argue that all the attention given to the development and provision of vaccines is really a diversion of attention from the real problems of health in poor countries. These demand much more radical efforts of an essentially socio-economic kind. A magic bullet approach is only a way of diverting attention from the real problems. This, too, is an issue that we have not gone into, and do not feel qualified to discuss.

What can be done?

W.P. Hausdorff (attached both to USAID and to a major manufacturer, Lederle) has recently made a number of interesting observations on this whole area (Hausdorff 1996). He argues that the economics of vaccine production do not necessarily make it unattractive to Northern manufacturers to supply vaccines at a price poor countries (or donor agencies) can afford, although it remains the case, according to him, that resources available are not sufficient to drive R&D programmes. The problem may be, in part, that the governments of poor countries have not always given vaccine supply, in the context of preventive health, a sufficiently high priority. He goes on to make two interesting proposals. The first is the need to explore new sources of revenue (for example, 'the large middle and upper classes in India who ... may be able to pay industrialized world prices for vaccines'). The second is the idea that the WHO define 'the characteristics of a specific priority vaccine which, if achieved, would then lead to a global recommendation for use'. Both these suggestions are intended to make the vaccines field more attractive to international pharmaceutical companies by increasing the likelihood of profit. Whether enhanced profitability of the vaccine field necessarily corresponds with the improvement of health is a matter on which not everyone is as yet agreed. From the point of view of a poor country, obliged to assume financial responsibility for an existing immunization programme within a limited health budget, international pressure to develop a new initiative could pose major problems.

In fact, a great deal has already been done, and it concerns not only financial resources. The journal *Science*, in its special section on vaccines entitled 'Bumps on the vaccine road' (Science 1994), dealt with many of the obstacles in the way of bringing needed vaccines to the populations of developing countries. 'The absence of strong market incentives', explains one author, 'increases the need for effective leadership from public-sector organizations devoted to vaccine development' (Cohen 1994: 1372). At the political level a number of initiatives have indeed been taken. The best known and most visible of these recent initiatives is the Children's Vaccine Initiative.

Behind the initiation of the CVI in 1991 lay a widespread concern with the degree of fragmentation – or disarticulation – of vaccine development: disarticulation between basic research work, development work, and delivery in the field (Muraskin 1996, 1996a). The development stage in particular is problematic because of the growing dominance of commercial considerations. (The role of public sector agencies is being undermined, with privatization and 'consolidation' of the vaccine industry. Vaccines are said to be in the process of becoming 'just another form of commercial merchandise'). The principal impetus, however, was less the drive to coordinate all of this than 'to exert a greater public sector influence over the product development part of the process'.

What followed seems to have been a process of political coalition forming, in which a variety of actors sought to align their very different interests around a concept which could generate high level political support. In the process, the concept changed quite dramatically. The starting point seems to have been D.A. Henderson's proposal for a 'Manhattan-type project' aimed at improving the stability and efficacy of polio vaccine (1989). UNICEF then broadened the idea enormously – beyond what Henderson thought reasonable – in order partly to justify the organisation's moving into the R&D area. The 'single vaccine' idea is a further modification of the initial concept, thought to be a suitable 'rallying cry' around which the scientific community could mobilize. The form of the initiative, including its later transformation from the search for a Children's Vaccine to an 'Initative', as well as the subsequent involvement of WHO, seems to have everything to do with effective coalition-building. The initiative should capture the attention of world leaders, represent an acceptable step back from the 'unrealistic' Alma Ata declaration, and reassert a degree of political control over the (commercialized) vaccine development process.

Four years later, *Science* found very mixed opinions regarding what the CVI had achieved and was likely to achieve. Some scientists and policymakers involved were concerned by lack of leadership, whilst others pointed to new combination vaccines which had emerged from the initiative (Gibbons 1994: 1376). Most recently, CVI seems – from the documents – to have information exchange, development of networks of researchers, manufacturers and planners, gaining commitment to immunization initiatives, and (a matter of seeming disagreement) developing capacity in poor countries among its principal goals.

The CVI is, in fact, only the most visible of a number of initiatives and developments which have begun to transform the vaccines field. I am not going to provide an analysis of the transformation which is now taking place, since this is the subject of research which Ingrid Geesink and I are now carrying out in collaboration with Judith Justice. Suffice it to mention that among the most important factors underlying present developments have been the emergence of new techniques (based in molecular biology, genetics, immunology, protein chemistry) which have made totally new approaches to vaccine development – one might now speak of vaccine 'design' – possible. In the place of old approaches using killed or attenuated organisms, scientists now work with portions of those organisms, or of their DNA, which may have been produced wholly synthetically. With these new techniques, which have made many feel that some of the most difficult problems in vaccine development can be solved, have come new companies with specialized expertise in molecular biology.

New research techniques and new industrial interest are central to recent changes in the vaccine field. New political interest is also noticeable among the industrialised countries, provoked by fear of the re-emergence of old epidemic diseases and the emergence of new ones (see Kager, this volume). As vaccine 'design' moves back from the 'bush' (where it can draw on the long experience of clinicians familiar with norms, values, ways of life, prevalent understandings of disease) into the pristine laboratories of California's biotechnology companies, could something be lost? Is there a risk that the whole development process will be inadequately informed by knowledge of conditions in the field? That too is something we are trying to investigate. Opinion among experts with whom we have talked is that this is probably not a real danger. *Nature*'s recent 'briefing' on malaria outlines a number of new malaria vaccines now undergoing tests. All of these are synthetic, and many of them have been developed in biotechnology companies (Nature 1997: 537-8).

These developments have also sparked new interest among the major pharmaceutical companies whose expertise and resources will be essential if the new synthetic vaccines are to be produced and tested in large-scale clinical trials. New collaborations, new alignments, new commitments are being made by some of the world's largest pharmaceutical companies. Some firms which had totally left the vaccine field are now reconsidering. In Europe, the pharmaceutical companies that do make vaccines have established the European Vaccine Manufacturers under the aegis of the European Pharmaceutical Manufacturer's Association, and this EVM has been politically active. It has sponsored a number of European conferences on 'vaccinology' and sought harmonization of trials and regulations within Europe. The European Union has established a Task Force on Vaccines. It is difficult to tell what the effects of all this will be on the work of developing vaccines, still less on meeting the immunization needs of children and adults in the developing world.

We have to look carefully at how these new alignments, and the rhetoric of Geneva, New York and Brussels, affects what really goes on. For example, in what ways is the scientific and technological capacity of vaccine institutes *in* poor countries being enhanced (Bloom 1989)? Is their capacity to manufacture existing vaccines under licence according to industrialized country standards of good manufacturing practice being enhanced? Perhaps so. Some vaccines researchers see:

an enormous shift in vaccines research and production, to Taiwan, Korea, India. A great deal is going on in Asia. We'll miss the boat if we don't try to go along with that. One problem with technology transfer is that the techniques for vaccine development can also be used for making biological weapons... (Osterhaus 1997).

Other issues arise. In how far are clinical trials of candidate vaccines sensitive to social and cultural features of the trial populations? How is the changing political economy of vaccines affecting the choices being made in industry? For example, it appears that differences in immunocompetence mean that children in developing countries typically have less benefit from existing measles vaccines than those in developed countries. A different vaccine may be needed (Spier 1993: 1451). Who chooses to direct their efforts in that direction rather than an improved measles vaccine for use in the developed world? There is a great need for interdisciplinary studies (like Tandon's study of leprosy vaccine and Viswanath's of anti-fertility vaccine, both being developed at the Indian Institute of Immunology) which combine insights from medical anthropology, sociology of science and political economy.

Notes

1 Thus, de Quadros of the Pan American Health Organisation, writes 'The simplicity of the vaccine and its mode of administration was critical to the campaign's final success in 1977. The smallpox vaccine was highly heat stable and did not require refrigeration in the field, and only one dose conferred protection. Health workers with relatively little training could administer the vaccine...' (De Quadros et al. 1994).

2 It seems that on average the costs of cold chain maintenance approximate the costs of vaccine purchase: approximately 8% of the costs of vaccinating a child in a developing country. EPI vaccines differ substantially in terms of their thermal stability, from the relatively stable DPT to the relatively unstable oral polio and measles vaccines.

3 Peter Beverley, an immunologist and director of Britain's new Edward Jenner Institute for Vaccine Research, suggests that 'the bigger the genome, the less successful we've been'. Contrast successful development of antiviral vaccines with the continuing failure to develop successful vaccines against parasitic diseases (Beverley 1997).

4 RIVM has made technology transfer, and assisting vaccines institutes in developing countries to develop and produce vaccines according to the highest standards of gmp a major plank in its strategy. See RIVM, n.d.

5 See Desowitz (1991). According to a recent analysis of malaria research, approximately 12% of scientific papers dealing with malaria report studies of vaccine trials, vaccine development and immunological responses. Approximately the same proportion of papers report studies of drug discovery and development. See Anderson, MacLean and Davies 1996; Tandon, 1996. Brian Greenwood, an experienced parasitologist and long-time director of the MRC Research Unit in The Gambia, suggests that this opposition is specific to these two diseases (Greenwood 1997).

6 Children under 10 had been excluded from the first published analyses.

7 One at least failed, and the resulting 'Cutter incident' had major repercussions. See, for example, Gould 1995, Chapter 6.

8 For discussion of some of the specifics of AIDS vaccine trials see Grady 1995.

9 Calculations suggested that even with efficacies of 30-50% (though some estimated 0%!), and assuming a 5-year protection period, a vaccine could save lots of lives. The lower the efficacy and the shorter the duration of protection, the greater the cost of an immunization programme. Preliminary estimates based on mathematical models suggest that in areas of blanket transmission, the best approach is 'blanket coverage of the sexually active population, repeated annually in an unselective manner' ... the cost is likely to be extremely high.

10 It is perhaps worth noting that even in Western industrialized cultures the concept of 'informed consent' – implying a rational individual actor – has come under criticism. Some have denied that this conceptualization does justice to the social processes, involving consultation in a family, which are often involved in consenting to an experimental procedure. See Kuczewski 1996.

Literature

Anderson, J., M. MacLean & C. Davies
   1996   *Malaria research*. PRISM Unit report No. 7. London: Wellcome Trust.
Basch, P.
   1994   *Vaccines and world health*. New York: OUP.
Beverley, P.
   1997   Interview with the author, Compton, June.
Bloom B.R.
   1989   'Vaccines for the Third World.' *Nature* 342: 115-120.
Blume, S.S.
   1992   *Insight and industry: the dynamics of technological change in medicine.* Cambridge Mass: MIT Press.
   1995   'Cochlear implantation: Establishing clinical feasibility, 1957-1982.' In: N. Rosenberg, A.C. Gelijns & H. Dawkins (eds), *Sources of medical technology*. Washington DC: National Academy of Sciences Press, pp. 97-124.

Brandt, A.M.
    1978   'Polio, politics, publicity and duplicity: Ethical aspects in the development
            of the Salk vaccine.' *International Journal of Health Services* 8: 257-70.
Cohen, J.
    1994   'Bumps on the vaccine road.' *Science* 265: 1371-3.
De Quadros, C.A., J-M. Olive & P. Carrasco
    1994   'The desired field-performance characteristics of new improved vaccines
            for the developing world.' *International Journal of Technology Assess-
            ment in Health Care* 10: 65-70.
Desowitz, R.S.
    1991   *The malaria capers.* New York: W.W. Norton.
Eickhoff, T.C.
    1988   'Bacille Calmette-Guerin (BCG) vaccine.' In: S. Plotkin & E.A. Mortimer
            (eds), *Vaccines.* Philadelphia: W.B. Saunders, pp. 372-386.
Epstein, S.
    1995   'The construction of lay expertise: AIDS activism and the forging of credi-
            bility in the reform of clinical trials.' *Science Technology & Human Values*
            20: 408-437.
Fenner, F., D.A. Henderson, I. Arita, Z. Jezek & I.D. Ladnyi
    1988   *Smallpox and its eradication.* Geneva: WHO.
Fine, P.E.M.
    1989   'The BCG story: Lessons from the past and implications for the future.'
            Reviews of Infectious Diseases 11 (Supplement 2): S357.
Gibbons, A.
    1994   'Childrens' Vaccine Initiative stumbles.' *Science* 265: 1376-7.
Gould, T.
    1995   *A summer plague: Polio and its survivors.* New Haven and London: Yale
            University Press.
Grady, C.
    1995   *The search for an AIDS Vaccine.* Bloomington Ind: Indiana University Press.
Greenwood, B.
    1997   *Interview with the author*, London, June.
Hausdorff, W.P.
    1996   'Prospects for the use of new vaccines in developing countries: cost is not
            the only impediment.' *Vaccine* 14: 1179-86.
Institute of Medicine
    1986   *New vaccine development: Establishing priorities.* Vol. 2. Washington DC:
            National Academy Press.
Kuczewski, M.G.
    1996   'Reconceiving the family: the process of consent in medical decision-
            making.' *Hastings Center Report* 26: 30-37.

McLean, A.A., E.B. Buynak, B.J. Kuter, M.R. Hilleman & D.J. West
  1984   'Clinical experience with Hepatitis B vaccine.' In: I. Millman, T.K. Eisen-
         stein & B.S. Blumberg (eds), *Hepatitis B: The virus, the disease and the
         vaccine.* New York: Plenum Press.

Millman, I.
  1984   'The development of the hepatitis B vaccine.' In: I. Millman, T.K. Eisen-
         stein & B. Blumberg (eds), *Hepatitis B: The virus, the disease and the
         vaccine.* New York: Plenum Press, pp. 137-147.

Mitchell, V.S., N.M. Philipose & J.P. Sanford (eds)
  1993   *The Children's Vaccine Initiative: Achieving the vision.* Washington DC:
         National Academy Press.

Moore, J. & R. Anderson
  1994   'The WHO and why of HIV vaccine trials.' *Nature* 372: 313-4.

Moxon, R.E.
  1990   'The scope of immunisation.' *Lancet* 448-451.

Muraskin, W.
  1996   'Origins of the Children's Vaccine Initiative: The intellectual founda-
         tions.' *Social Science and Medicine* 42(12): 1703-1719.

  1996a 'Origins of the Children's Vaccine Initiative: The political foundations.'
         Social Science and Medicine 42(12): 1721-1734.

Nature
  1997   'Vaccines: a roller-coaster of hopes.' *Nature* 386: 537-538.

Osterhaus, A.D.M.E.
  1997   Interview with I. Geesink, Rotterdam, August.

Petricciani, J.C., V.P. Grachev, P.P. Sizaret & P.J. Regan
  1989   'Vaccines: obstacles and opportunities from discovery to use.' *Reviews of
         Infectious Diseases* 11 (Supplement 3): S524-529.

Rijksinstituut voor Volksgezondheid en Milieuhygiene (RIVM)
  n.d.   *International Vaccine Policy.* Bilthoven: RIVM.

Science
  1994   *Number 265.*

Spier, R.E.
  1993   'Conference Report: Meeting on Vaccine Strategies for Tomorrow.' *Vac-
         cine* 11: 1450-52.

Tandon, S.
  1996   *A sociological study fo the development of anti-leprosy vaccines.* Social
         Science and Immunisation Country Study: India. Working paper. Delhi:
         Centre for Development Economics.

Viswanath, K. & P. Kirbat
  1996   *Recent developments in fertility regulating vaccines in India.* Social Scien-
         ce and Immunization Country Study: India. Working paper. Delhi: Centre
         for Development Economics.

CHAPTER IX

From the Bench to the Bush:
The Development of a Diagnostic Test

Wiepko Terpstra & Henk Smits

The problem

In the industrialized Northern countries our daily life is unthinkable without products from technology, like the telephone, television, cars, electric light and clean, piped water. Much research goes into achieving good and safe products. Researcher workers in laboratories may come up with results that appear valuable for application. However, there is a long road to go from the result on the workbench of the researcher to the final product for the consumer. We do not always realize that each applicable technical tool is the end result of a painstakingly precise and detailed process. On the way to large-scale manufacture, each aspect of the new tool has been scrutinized, improved and worked on to make a reliable product. Take, for example, diagnostics.

Diagnostics are tools to make or help make a diagnosis, for instance, to find out whether a patient has an infection or not. Diagnostics are needed because many diseases lack characteristic clinical manifestations, and it may be difficult or sometimes even impossible for the clinician to make a diagnosis on clinical grounds only. Such a diagnosis is crucial when a disease is dangerous and its outcome can be influenced by carefully attuned intervention, for instance, with a certain kind of antibiotic. In addition, a diagnosis is important if recognition of the disease may have public health impact, for instance in case of an outbreak that would otherwise go unnoticed, but needs to be contained.

For this contribution we add the additional difficulty of application in the bush. If the road from the bench to application in affluent and sophisticated industrialized countries is already long and complicated, think how difficult it is to transform a good piece of work in the laboratory into a reliable well-functioning test in the tropical bush. To give an example: many diagnostics contain reagents that are unstable, that just like food need to be preserved, e.g. in a refrigerator. Or, to perform a test, an apparatus may be needed which requires electricity. The availability of such a supportive environment may be a necessary condition for the proper application of the diagnostic tool.

The dilemmas of the industry and of Northern funding agencies

Pharmaceutical industries have already been producing all kinds of diagnostic tests for a long time. But health professionals who are interested in tropical diseases, or involved in their control, frequently lack appropriate tests. This is because industries are often not interested in their production, as they fear high investment costs and scant financial returns.

Similarly, Dutch or international agencies that provide funding for health research may not put tropical diseases high on their priority list. There are plenty of health problems in industrialized Northern countries such as heart diseases, cancer, rheumatoid arthritis and diseases related to old age which compete for funding. Even though tropical diseases are scientifically interesting, they do not score high in terms of public health. Since other health problems are perceived as more pressing, research on tropical diseases remains in a comparatively backward situation. This situation not only applies to relatively rare tropical diseases, but also to diseases like malaria, which occur frequently in the tropics and cause important health problems. For a disease like HIV/AIDS, which is also a health problem in the North, the situation is a bit different: this disease receives substantial funding for research.

One may compare tropical diseases to orphans, left alone with nobody taking loving care of them. This neglect may also mean that the means or tools to detect these diseases are lacking. Consequently, even in countries where certain diseases occur, doctors and patients may not or may only dimly be aware that these diseases are causing them harm.

The Royal Tropical Institute's (KIT) Department of Biomedical Research (BO) is interested in research on infectious diseases causing health problems in the tropics, which can crudely and ineptly be described as tropical diseases. The department is interested in methods and tools to detect these diseases and, once these tools have been developed, in how to use them to collect information about these diseases, on where they occur, how often they occur, how they are transmitted, and how their transmission can be interrupted.

How BO's research experience evolved

For a long time BO has been involved in the development of diagnostic tests. The development of such tests was an aim in itself. It was an intellectual and scientific challenge to make a test that performed well under the harsh conditions of the bush. Additionally, once developed, it was intriguing to find out how these tests performed in efforts to investigate health problems, clinical as well as public health ones.

BO has made its knowledge and skills, including those to perform tests, available to partners in developing countries and has transferred its knowledge in training courses and publications. So far, BO has introduced many tests all over the world and taught how to interpret the results, thus contributing to the creation of local centres of expertise in the South. The idea was that, once these skills and knowledge had been transferred, they would gradually spread into the periphery of the countries concerned. There was definitely a spreading effect, but in the sense that more and related technology geared to control of other diseases was gathered and adopted in the same place. Spreading to the periphery also took place, it is true, but this should have occurred faster.

Technologies which are considered basic in the North are sometimes deemed complex by the standards of staff who have to work with them in institutes and health centres in developing countries. To adjust to this problem, we took the decision to go one step further and make diagnostic tools that combine extreme simplicity with reliability so that the technology could spread more easily from local centres to the periphery. This was an additional challenge: transferring not from the bench in the North to the bench in the South, but from the bench in the North to the bush in the South. Unavoidably and consciously, in this way we decided on an industrial approach, as such an aim implies the production of very large numbers of tests.

Over the years BO has developed satisfactory ties of collaboration with pharmaceutical companies. So far, this industry has not shown signs of wanting to commercially exploit the tests that were generated by BO over the past few years. When KIT provided funds to BO to take action on its own to explore commercial applications, BO designed and developed tests into formats that approached commercial products, prototypes, manufactured but not yet in large numbers.[1]

The Department of Biomedical Research was exploring opportunities that have not been self-evident, to turn scientists into entrepreneurs making use of skills and knowledge that were acquired during many years of experience with more basic research. BO is now facing a situation in which a scientist must adopt the attitude of an entrepreneur who has to deal with customers. This is mentality-wise a complete turnabout. To express it in an exaggerated way, the essentially non-committal contemplative attitude of the scientist must be transformed into the fully committed attitude of the practical worker that matter-of-factly deals with the cold and uncompromising realities of a product and its consumer.

BO's experience was mainly in the field of serology, i.e. the detection in a person's blood of antibodies directed against a certain pathogen. The finding of such antibodies means that the patient is either at that very moment infected with the pathogen or has been infected in the past. Serology involves, in other words, finding indirect evidence of a current, recent or past infection. The emphasis is on the word indirect as not the pathogen itself is detected but the patient's reaction to the pathogen. Mounting an immune response, i.e. production of antibodies by a person, takes some time, and the immune response wanes gradually over weeks, months or years. There is considerable difference between pathogens, and immune responses may differ between patients. Another important point is that the reliability of serological tests has limitations. This is well-known and accepted and is related to a variety of defined and undefined factors such as duration of the disease, differences between patients' immune responses, previous infections, other infections and so on. The reliability of tests is usually expressed in terms of sensitivity and specificity, as a percentage.

For all these reasons, tests based on serology are an approximation, and their results should be considered as an adjunct to the clinical differential diagnosis based on signs and symptoms, clinical and epidemiological history, or other sources of information.

The long road to the product

The process from bench to product and, eventually, to the bush can be described in the following series of steps: conception leads to research leads to development leads to evaluation leads to production leads to marketing and distribution. When one considers making a product, it is unavoidable that from the outset all the aspects in the chain of steps mentioned above must be considered in detail. In other words, careful planning is essential as later on, when the process of production has started to roll, it gains a lot of momentum and by then it is difficult and costly to change direction.

Research should of course be planned and laid out in a schedule of sequential activities, but serendipity, which is by definition unplanned, is sometimes of crucial importance. In any case, one should be alert for promising findings in research. Flexibility in research is good, and re-adjustment of adapted research plans may be desirable. However, as stated earlier, once one has embarked on the road towards production, deviation is next to impossible.

Before we consider the steps involved in more detail by focussing on the example of the development of a diagnostic tool for *leptospirosis*, let us consider the key issues of markets and products.

In the case of a problem of tropical diseases that needs to be diagnosed, there is a demand but not necessarily a strong market. The market is probably weak because these diseases are mainly found in developing countries with economically poor populations. When these diseases are found in Northern industrialised countries, they are usually rare, and consequently, tests are only infrequently required. Besides, as mentioned above, international pharmaceutical companies are not interested in developing and producing diagnostics for tropical diseases because of the doubtful prospect that the investments will be adequately returned. However, there might be a niche for small entrepreneurs who work at relatively low expense levels. Moreover, the outlook for return of investments may after all not be so bleak as often thought, because the economies in many tropical countries are growing rapidly, and some of the populations are increasingly able to pay, modestly perhaps, for health care.

Given such a market situation, the conditions which a product, in this case a diagnostic tool, must fulfil can be described as follows. In principle, availability of a minimum of equipment to perform tests is desirable, but the ideal test should not need any additional equipment. In view of the requirement that our diagnostic test must perform in the bush, its stability and simplicity will be strongly emphasized. The price should be low, at least affordable. The test must be simple enough to be performed by basically trained personnel. It must be of a standard quality: the same results are obtained with test kits used by different hands in different areas under different conditions. The test must be of good quality, specific and sensitive and in addition reliable, giving within its range of application trustworthy results that contribute greatly to the clinician's ability to make a diagnosis. The test reagents must be stable so that they retain their activity even under adverse conditions, notably high temperatures. This is because in tropical countries cold chains for storage and distribution are expensive, and refrigerators, if available, may not always function optimally due to frequent power failures. Since short expiry dates mean frequent, laborious and costly replacements of expired test kits, they must have a long shelf-life, meaning that if adequately stored they can be kept in good condition for a long time.

The product must be backed-up by a good service, which includes that the distributor has sufficient items in stock to rapidly satisfy consumer demand. Consumers must have a name and address to send questions and complaints to. The packaging of the tools must be convenient for storage and handling of the contents. The package must be resistant to rather 'rough' conditions. The packing must contain an easy to understand insert explaining what procedures must be followed to perform a test and how to interpret the test results. These procedures should be similar to those required to perform other tests so that even basically trained personnel will be familiar with them.

The case of *leptospirosis*

We shall now describe the stepwise development of a product, using the example of a diagnostic tool to detect whether a person suffers from the disease *leptospirosis*. The disease, with its better known variety Weil's disease, occurs worldwide but quite often in humid tropical countries. The doctors usually rely heavily on the laboratory for support for their clinical suspicion as there are many other diseases that are very similar to *leptospirosis*, e.g. so-called haemorrhagic fevers, a group of diseases in which the patient has a tendency to bleed. An outbreak of a 'bleeding disease' in Nicaragua two years ago turned out eventually to be leptospirosis. It is important to know whether a patient suffers from leptospirosis or not because in a positive case adequate treatment with antibiotics should be started without delay.

A very important issue to be faced by BO is that, for quality assurance, tests must be produced according to stringent rules and standards that are set by national and international authorities. Producing according to good manufacturing practice (GMP) is a prerequisite. For products for veterinary use, registration, i.e. a procedure in which permission is obtained to deal in the product, is already a necessity, while for human diagnostics the obligation to register is expected to be introduced within a few years. Producing according to GMP is costly, and BO cannot afford to fully implement it on its own; BO must collaborate with the pharmaceutical industry. New regulations are in the pipeline, and it remains to be seen how, for instance, European regulations apply to sales in the tropics.

Another consideration concerns the cost of the process of developing and producing the test. In fact, all expenses ranging from salaries to chemicals, purchase of equipment, maintenance of the laboratory, etc., involving the whole process from conception to distribution should be covered, and a 'profit' should be generated that allows, at least in KIT's option, the continuation of research by BO.

Conception

The conventional methods for diagnosis of this disease in the laboratory are difficult to perform. We aimed at the development of a method that would allow diagnosis even under difficult circumstances. We designed a dipstick-like type of test. In this test, a little bit of a reagent which is called antigen is extracted from micro-organisms that we call *leptospires* cultured in the laboratory. This antigen attached to a teststrip is glued to the end of a plastic stick the size of a match. Blood, or rather serum, of the patient is mixed with a developer reagent in a tube. The teststrip of the stick is dipped in the tube. If the patient has antibodies, indicating exposure to the micro-organism, this will show by a red staining of the antigen: antibodies react with the antigen and the developing reagent reveals this by a red stain on the teststrip at the place where the antigen now covered with antibodies is located. The concept sounds simple enough.

Research

After a plan had been formulated, a research programme was initiated to work out a test. We made various types of extracts (antigens) of the micro-organism, the *leptospires*, in order to find out which type of antigen is good in binding antibodies. Some antigens are too weak; one hardly sees a stain. Others are too strong; one sees red staining when it should not be there, because the patient has antibodies but to micro-organisms other than *leptospires*. In brief, after countless attempts finally a good way to extract antigen was found. And so on, meaning that all the different reagents and components of the dipstick were prepared after numerous time-consuming tests.

If research is successful and leads to new findings, patenting should be considered. Patents are expensive to obtain and may be expensive to protect. The dipstick had already been patented by a pharmaceutical company, and BO acquired a license agreement for its further development and production.

Development

This step is actually still part of the research phase and aims at developing a prototype. In this case the emphasis was on bringing all the different components together in one format, that is a dipstick. All components were carefully tuned to each other so that the reaction chain led to a balanced and easily readable result. A moderately large number of dipsticks were produced in the laboratory according to a standardized procedure.

Evaluation[2]

The test is first evaluated within the walls of the laboratory to establish its efficacy. This efficacy is usually expressed in terms of sensitivity and specificity which reflect the reliability of the test in detecting a disease. Then the test is distributed in a preferably prospective multicentre study in many places all over the world to check on its sensitivity and specificity in the hands of other people.

When tested within our own laboratory, we got results with the dipsticks that were at least as good as the difficult conventional tests. We found, in addition, that the dipsticks gave the same results day after day. Next, we distributed dipsticks widely around to many other laboratories elsewhere in the world asking them to test the dipstick and to compare it with their standard conventional tests. In some of these laboratories, prospective studies were initiated to test the dipstick on every sample of all patients suspected of having the disease. So far, the results have been satisfactory, with few discrepancies. The discrepancies are being investigated; first of all, we are looking into the kind of test that is routinely applied and used as the gold standard by the laboratory in question.

Production, marketing and distribution

The step from prototype to product involves upscaling production of the product to industrial proportions while maintaining the same quality standard in each item. Rigorous standardisation is thus required for every single step in the production process and careful quality control before, during and at the end of the production process. Marketing addresses the potential customers. To this end the customers must be identified, localised and quantified, or at least their numbers must be estimated. It must be clear to the customers why they should buy the test. For less well-known diseases awareness must be raised as test consumers may not know that there is a problem. Through promotion it must be made evident that there is an actual, but hidden need. Potential customers may not know that there is a solution, at least a diagnostic solution, for their problem. So the product awareness must be created, increased or stimulated by advertisements, workshops, papers, mailings and sending of free specimens. Actually, from the very beginning one should have an idea of whether the intended product has an added value over possible competing products, and during promotion campaigns the advantages of the product in comparison with the competitor's product should be emphasised. Of course this includes careful setting of a price. Adequate stocks of products with a sufficiently long shelf-life and a flexible production process must be maintained in order to be able to meet sudden changes in demands. Distributing agencies in different countries must have good transport and storage facilities.

For all this, we are now seeking the help of the pharmaceutical industry, because BO itself does not have the necessary capabilities. As for marketing, it is important to know how many patients contract *leptospirosis*, in certain areas, or even worldwide. This is hard to know exactly because almost by definition little is known about a neglected disease like leptospirosis. In some Northern countries we have reasonably good indications of how often the disease occurs. We know that it strikes in tropical countries, but in many areas we do not know how often, while for some areas we can make an educated guess. We guess rather than estimate that the number of cases worldwide is approximately 200,000 per year. However, there is obviously some uncertainty about the size of the market.

Furthermore BO intends to explore the possibility of setting up collaborative activities if not joint ventures with partners in the tropics. The department realises that entering this field demands care as entrepreneurial issues such as secrecy, patents and intellectual property must be considered. These issues may be experienced by some as contradictory to the perhaps old-fashioned and superseded if not naive spirit of freedom of science with access to all new developments for everybody. The spirit of free enterprise demands a calculating mind and an open eye for developments with a promise of profit which requires a certain reversal of attitude for many traditional scientists.

BO hopes for a situation which is beneficial for all partners involved: BO can continue its research to contribute to health in the tropics, consumers of the tests benefit by making diagnoses that previously were impossible or impractical, and last but certainly not least, partners in the tropics may benefit by the transfer of skills and knowledge. In view of the demands of GMP partnership with the pharmaceutical industry is a necessity. Presently, many problems still remain that have to do with intellectual property and patenting, and with regulations and certifications required from governments.

Future potentials

In the tropics, there is a wide range of health problems caused by infectious diseases which are neglected. Some of these diseases have already been on BO's agenda for a long time. When developing diagnostic tools BO has aimed at the outset for the broadest possible applicability under conditions ranging from well-equipped central institutions to far away peripheral hospitals, even true field situations. Accordingly, some of BO's tests have been carried out in the open air under a tree. To allow field use BO has also designed its tests from the outset to be stable and durable, enabling them to withstand the rigours of the tropics.

We now shall conclude by giving some examples of other, less well-known diseases for which BO has developed diagnostic tests. *Visceral leishmaniasis* is a serious lethal disease which affects worldwide an estimated 200,000-500,000 patients per year, a.o. in India, Bangladesh and Sudan. BO has developed a so-called agglutination test. This test is based on the principle that the antibodies in a patient's blood make the so-called antigen, in this case specially preserved pathogens, clump to form aggregates that can be observed with the naked eye. The test is commercially available, but the marketing has not yet had much success. The test is being subject to further simplification.

BO has already produced a dipstick which rapidly detects antibodies to *leptospires* as described above. A dipstick to detect antibodies to *Salmonella typhi*, the pathogen that causes typhoid, is in the process of being evaluated. The current serological tests for typhoid are not considered satisfactory. An estimated 16,000,000 cases of typhoid, a potentially fatal disease, occur each year worldwide.

Attention has also been paid to the development of a similar dipstick test for the serodiagnosis of *brucellosis*, an often severe disease which is transmitted to humans from cattle, goats and pigs by ingestion of raw milk, milk-products or contact with other animal materials. The disease is caused by infection by, respectively, *Brucella abortus*, B. melitensis and B. *suis*. *Brucellosis* exists worldwide, especially in countries of the Mediterranean basin, the Arabian Gulf, the Indian subcontinent, and parts of Mexico and Central and South America. Six countries in the Middle East reported together 90,000 cases a year.

BO also developed a dipstick for leprosy, a disease with 500,000 new cases each year. The immune response in this disease is complicated. Test results must be carefully considered in relation to the patient's clinical presentation. The leprosy dipstick is under evaluation. It may turn out that this dipstick is suitable for population studies, to find out about the occurrence of leprosy in general, and also for the benefit of the individual patient.

In the tropics, basic information on incidence, mortality and morbidity is lacking for many diseases. In fact, had there been reliable data, then the tools to gather these data would already have been available, and there would have been little incentive to make new tools. Plans for the production and marketing of tests must be made, but there is a dilemma, as solid figures on which to base these plans are lacking. From the commercial interest to pursue guaranteed gains this is perhaps an unattractive situation. Going from the bench to the bush means entering unexplored territory. There is an unavoidable risk involved. Exploring, however, is highly intriguing to the daring.

Notes

1 As for the term 'commercially', to prevent misunderstanding it should be stressed that the KIT is a non-profit organisation that works on a cost-recovery basis and does not make profits.

2 Evaluations were possible thanks to collaboration with colleagues and organisations working in the field, notably 'Doctors without Frontiers', but BO is indebted to many more supporters.

Literature

Bankowski Z. & G.L. Ada

1989

Health Technology Transfer: Whose responsibility? Paper for the xxiiird CIOMS Round Table Conference, Geneva, Switzerland, 2-3 November 1989.

Gussenhoven G.C., M.A.W.G. Van der Hoorn, M.G.A. Goris, W.J. Terpstra, R.A. Hartskeerl, B.W. Mol. C.W. Van Ingen & H.L. Smits

1997 'LEPTO dipstick, a distick assay for detection of *Leptospira*-specific immunoglobulin M antibodies in human sera.' *J Clin Microbiol* 35: 92-97.

Oskam L., R.J. Slappendel, E.G.M. Beijer, N.C.M. Kroon & C.W. van Ingen, S. Özensoy, Y. Özbel & W.J. Terpstra

1996 'Dog-DAT: A direct agglutination test using stabilized, freeze-dried antigen for the serodiagnosis of canine visceral leishmaniasis.' *FEMS Immunol Med Microbiol* 16: 235-239.

Meredith S.E.O., C.C.M. Kroon, E. Sondorp, J. Seaman, M.G.A. Goris, C.W. van Ingen, H. Oosting, G.J. Schoone, W.J. Terpstra & L. Oskam

1995 '*Leish*-KIT, a stable direct agglutination test based on freeze-dried antigen for serodiagnosis of visceral leishmaniasis.' *J Clin Microbiol* 33: 1742-1745.

World Health Organization

1996 *The World Health Report 1996. Fighting disease, fostering development.* Geneva: WHO.

1997 *The World Health Report 1997. Conquering suffering, enriching humanity.* Geneva: WHO.

CHAPTER X

Use and Misuse of Pharmaceuticals: Anthropological Comments

SJAAK VAN DER GEEST[1]

In 1984 a mother in a Filipino village took her child to a doctor. The child had diarrhoea. The doctor prescribed five medicines, the total cost of which equalled one week's salary. Hardon (1987), who reported this case, comments that it was an ordinary diarrhoea which could have been treated with a simple salt solution. It would have cost her nearly nothing. The doctor, however, prescribed an anti-vomit medicine, an anti-diarrhoea medicine, an antibiotic, a multivitamin product and a painkiller. The prescription was harmful, not only in a financial sense (waste of money) but also medically; the anti-diarrhoea medicine contained a substance which should not be given to children below the age of three.

Senah, who did field work in a coastal village in Ghana, provides the following case of a woman called Dedei:

Dedei had been complaining of persistent bodily weakness, headache, cold, catarrh, and feeling feverish. She diagnosed her problem as malaria and began to treat it accordingly. For four days, she took two tablets of chloroquine each morning, afternoon and evening. These tablets were purchased from the village drug store. When her condition did not improve, her husband advised her to take a combination of *Fansidar* and camoquine – two tablets each morning, afternoon and evening. However, a few days later, Dedei's friend advised that Dedei's ailment was in fact a new form of malaria popularly known as 'Go-slow' and that the medication for this was a concoction of pharmaceuticals popularly known as 'Mixture'. Dedei quickly procured this. As I learned later, Mixture is obtained from a combination of tetracycline and penicillin capsules, B-COMPLEX, chloroquine tablets and *Valium*. A few days later, when Dedei's problem persisted, she finally went to the hospital. Later, I was informed, she had been admitted with *asratriddii* (jaundice). She recovered after about three weeks (Senah 1994: 96).

In her study of long-term benzodiazepine use by 50 women in The Netherlands, Haafkens (1997: 57) describes the case of a woman who at the age of 23 became an unwed mother:

> When she was one month pregnant with her second child, at the age of 25, the father with whom she was living suddenly died in a traffic accident. Three months after the baby was born, she was given a daily dosage of 10 milligrams of benzodiazepam because she could not sleep... She was afraid of losing the custody over her children if she showed any weakness to professional helpers, or for that matter to any outsider, and did not dare to discuss her anger and sadness about the death of her boyfriend with anyone. She wanted to be 'one of those rare unwed mothers who was not making a mess of her life, and who could be a role model for an article in "Parents Today"', which is a Dutch journal on child raising. Soon after she got her first benzodiazepines, she felt benzodizapines were helping her to achieve this. She began to take a higher dosage every six weeks. Like her problems she did not want to discuss her benzediazepines with anyone either, not even with close friends: 'I was avoiding people, because they might discover I was taking pills. I pushed people away. Looking back, I avoided outsiders because I didn't want to admit to myself that I was taking pills.'

During my own research on birth control in a Ghanaian rural community, I came across many instances of self-medication for the purpose of abortion. Overdoses of anti-malaria pills or painkillers were some of the favourite ones. The following case involves another pharmaceutical. A young woman:

> After my first child I became pregnant again. The child was still very young and I did not want to have another child so soon, so I decided to remove it. My husband agreed. The pregnancy was only one month old. I took six *Alophen* pills, three consecutive days two pills, and after four days it came. Much blood came with it, but it was later that I felt sick and went to the clinic for treatment (Bleek 1978: 108).[2]

These four cases present four very different examples of dubious medicine use. In the first case, we see a medical doctor who makes a mother buy an expensive but quite useless prescription to treat a simple diarrhoea. The context of this incident is dominated by an incompetent and uncertain medical practitioner with a commercial attitude toward pharmaceuticals. By increasing the amount of prescribed medicines the doctor increases his confidence and income. The poor mother trusts him and makes a double mistake: she is wasting her precious money and runs the risk of causing medical harm to her child.

The second case portrays people outside the formal sector of health care, in a Ghanaian household. People without medical training, but with extensive practical experience, discuss the sickness of one of them. They take decisions which imply the use of several pharmaceuticals, which are purchased in a local drugstore. These medications are quite irrational from a biomedical point of view, but make sense to them. The context is the setting of a poor rural household, popular medical knowledge, and the absence of formal medical facilities.

The third example is situated in Dutch society where access to prescription medicines is strictly controlled, but where people still find ways to circumvent or cheat the gatekeepers to obtain the medicines to which they have become attached. Medical doctors are manipulated to achieve that goal. Once they have been prescribed tranquillisers, women are able to continue using them by having their first prescription renewed every time without the doctor checking this properly. The actual use of the medicines is carried out in secret. Doctors who prescribe the drugs lose track of them and join the women in an apparent conspiracy to avoid the topic of their (too) long use. Haafkens (1997: 148) concludes that most women she spoke with used the implicit rule 'Keep quiet about problems related to benzodiazepine use!' It demonstrates, in her words, 'the ambiguity of the very notion "prescription" drug.'

The last case is also an example of secrecy. The woman who wants to terminate her pregnancy is doing something which is publicly censored, but condoned in private. The main difference with the previous case is that the medicines which she applies are not meant to be used for that purpose. The context is characterised by medical ignorance, secrecy, and poverty; she cannot afford a safe abortion. No doctor is directly involved. The pills are bought in drugstores which operate largely outside the law.

Twenty years ago, when, as an anthropologist, I started to take an interest in the use of Western pharmaceuticals in 'non-Western' cultures, very little was known about this topic. There was one standard phrase which was copied over and over again in books and articles on health care in developing countries, namely that more than 70% of the population had no access to proper health care. By 'proper' was meant 'Western'.

During research in 1973 in Ghana, I had seen 'proper' pharmaceutical products in the most remote places I visited. Vermifuges, anti-malaria tablets, antibiotics and painkillers were being sold in small kiosks and from tables along the roadside. There was, however, hardly any sign of this phenomenon to be found in the literature.

A few years later, when I was making preparations for research on the distribution and use of pharmaceuticals in Cameroon, doctors who had worked there assured me that in Cameroon there was no selling of pharmaceuticals outside of hospitals or pharmacies. They must have been blind when they did their shopping at the local market. More likely, they never visited the market.

By now, we know that pharmaceuticals are indeed widely sold and used outside the formal medical context everywhere in the 'developing' world. Anthropologists and researchers from other disciplines have done valuable work to document these practices, but we are still grappling with a number of questions. Some of these are: How should we appreciate self-medication? How far does our understanding and acceptance of local medical rationalities go which clash head on with biomedical reason? Must we attempt to intervene to improve (according to our criteria) the quality of medicine use, and if so, how?

In this contribution I cannot tackle all these questions. The most difficult one, concerning rationality, I shall only touch upon. Although I am aware that there is more to pharmaceuticals than chemical-therapeutic substance, I shall here take the biomedical position on the dangers of pharmaceutical 'abuse'. Pharmaceuticals present a hard test to the anthropological doctrine of cultural respect and relativism. They are indeed charming examples of cultural creativity but the harm they produce is too evident to ignore.

I shall briefly sketch the cultural and infrastructural context of medicine use and then discuss three cultural processes which impinge on people's way of perceiving and taking pharmaceuticals. In the conclusion I shall offer some suggestions as to how the use of pharmaceuticals can be improved.

Throughout this paper I shall concentrate on situations in 'the South' which are most familiar to me, but, as Haafkens' research suggests, people in 'the North' are also busily engaged in self-medication practices which contradict biomedical precepts.

Supply of pharmaceuticals

Some years ago, a research team evaluating the WHO's Action Programme on Essential Drugs in a number of developing countries reported that they had not attempted to assess the implementation of the programme (Evaluation 1989, Kanji et al. 1992). By 'implementation' they meant making essential drugs available to the population. That question, they wrote, was too complex to be investigated within the allotted time and with the limited means available.

Although few exact data exist about the availability of pharmaceuticals in developing countries, some of the main problems of their supply have been extensively described and analysed (e.g. Melrose 1982, Silverman et al. 1982, Chetley 1990). These studies mention acute shortages of essential drugs and widespread inessential drugs. The authors attribute the situation to the dubious role of pharmaceutical companies and exporting countries as well as to bad management, irrational drug policy and lack of funds in the importing countries. To give an example, Chetley (1989: 5), who studied the marketing of cough and cold remedies in developing countries, reports that 91 such 'medicines' were being used in Africa and that almost half of them contained potentially harmful ingredients.

Most information on distribution deals with pharmaceuticals which are provided in hospitals and health centres.The situation in the informal market is still more chaotic. I counted 70 different drugs in a small Cameroonian town. A local physician gave as his opinion that 41 of them were useful and that 24 others should be withdrawn because of their risk. Asking how many of them could be classified as 'essential' made no sense because the information for correct use was not available from the person selling them. Wrongly used essential drugs can no longer be termed 'essential'. Ironically, more than half of the drugs the physician wanted to remove did indeed belong to the list of 'essential drugs' (Van der Geest 1987: 302-3). When we discuss the 'irrational' use of drugs, we should not lose sight of the fact that in most cases the medicines from which people have to choose constitute an irrational lot in themselves.

Use and misuse of pharmaceuticals

If so little is known about the supply of pharmaceuticals, what about their use? After all, rational use of drugs is the ultimate objective of the essential drugs programme. Kanji and Hardon (1992: 98) remark that 'despite the millions of dollars spent on formulating and implementing essential drugs policies world-wide, the impact of these activities depends a great deal on how rationally drugs are being used, and this has not been systematically evaluated.' Policy-makers and physicians often assume that once the proper drugs are available, people will use them in a correct and profitable way. That assumption, however, is overly optimistic. Studies of the use of antimalarial drugs, for example, show that even when the drugs can be obtained, proper use is not guaranteed. Foster (1991b, 1995) provides an overview of studies describing the problematic use patterns of antimalarials. Bleek (1978) and Senah (1997) report that antimalarials in Ghana are used to induce abortion.

Several case studies are now beginning to fill the blank spots of our knowledge of actual use of pharmaceuticals in developing countries. Hardon (1987, 1989) has produced valuable data on drugs use based on her fieldwork in both rural and urban communities in The Philippines. The results of a more recent four-country research project on community drug use are now appearing. Case studies of Uganda (Odoi Adome et al. 1996) and Pakistan (Rasmussen et al. 1996) have been published.[3] To give one example: in northern Pakistan 409 instances of medicine use were studied; 61% were found to be incorrect according to biomedical criteria (Rasmussen et al. 1996: 75).

We may still not have adequate data to make sound general statements about the use of pharmaceuticals in developing countries, but we do have sufficient fragmentary insights based on anthropological and other case studies to assemble some kind of overall picture. Two main impressions arise: 1) Modern pharmaceuticals are extremely popular among the majority of the population; and 2) their use by sick people is rarely guided by the medial profession. What drugs are being used is mainly determined by what drugs happen to be available, by people's financial possibilities and constraints, and by their perception of illness and drugs.

Popularity of pharmaceuticals

The 'pharmaceuticalization' of health and health care is a world-wide phenomenon, which is particularly pronounced in the developing world. Pharmaceuticals are seen as the essence of health care. Without them, the entire system loses its meaning. Health centres which run out of drugs also run out of patients. Medical treatment which does not include medication is nearly unthinkable. It is so in the eyes of the patients, and it has often also become the opinion of the health workers, who have learned otherwise. Community health workers lose their credibility as health educators when they have no drugs to dispense.

What has made pharmaceuticals so popular? Four aspects seem particularly relevant to answer that question. The first is that pharmaceuticals are tangible substances – a quality they share with 'traditional' medicines such as herbal drugs and amulets. Medicines are *things* which through their concreteness help people to come to grips with their health problems. They play a crucial role in making the inchoate experience of not feeling well graspable. Their concreteness is as it were contagious, they make concrete what is touched by them. The psychological relief brought about by a medical substance is that one can do some-*thing* against some-*thing*. This therapeutic reassurance is probably the main explanation for the universality of the use of substances in cases of illness (cf. Van der Geest & Whyte 1989).

Apart from this psychological factor, which applies to all types of medicines, modern pharmaceuticals have proved to be exceptionally effective. Antibiotics in particular have worked miracles in societies which were visited by a plethora of infectious diseases. The spectacular effects of injections added to the fame of Western pharmaceuticals (Wyatt 1984).

The 'power' of these medicines (Whyte 1988) is further increased by their foreign origin. Senah (1994) writes that pharmaceuticals in a coastal Ghanaian village are called *blofo tshofa* ('whiteman's medicine'). Things coming from afar are often considered to be better than those from home. Advertisements and packaging of drugs sometimes draw attention to this foreign origin by emphasizing their 'high tech' character (Tan 1989, 1996).

The aura of foreignness and high tech hovers especially around injections. More than any other pharmaceutical product, the injection demonstrates that it is from another world. Not the drug but the technical device by which it is administered forms the attraction (Reeler 1990, Bloem & Wolffers 1993). The injection is a metonym for the world of laboratories and scientific discoveries from whence so many other technical wonders originate. In some countries the needle and syringe have now become part of the medical self-help culture. Antibiotics, antimalarials, vitamins and other drugs are bought in drugstores and injected at home. The discussion below, which took place in a Ugandan shop, is a typical one:

A man came into a drug shop saying, ' have a patient at home who is bleeding too much.' The dresser who operated the shops asks: '... Do you have a syringe?' The customer affirms that he does and is sold a vial of injectable ergometrine and 15 flagyl tablets.

The fourth aspect of pharmaceuticals contributing to their popularity could be termed their 'liberating' effect. In local medical traditions, the quality of healers is usually seen as the decisive factor in therapeutic success. It is the healer who diagnoses the problem, finds and prepares the right medicines, and gives the medicine its power through prayer, ritual action, or otherwise. Medicines – and the entire therapeutic event – depend on the healer's art and intervention. African medical traditions are thus social systems par excellence. In periods of illness, people are forced to submit to others (elders, priests, medical specialists) to get rid of their problem. Sickness is an occasion for social control. Treatment and the working of medicines are linked to moral instructions.

Modern health care, however, is much more detached from the personal capacity of doctors and nurses. Western pharmaceuticals are seen as inherently therapeutic. Alland (1970: 170), who did research in the Ivory Coast, pointed out that people were not so much after the professional help of doctors or nurses but after pharmaceuticals. Doctors were seen as people one usually has to pass in order to get medicines. Having direct access to pharmaceuticals, in shops and marketplaces, was preferable.

Western pharmaceuticals allow people to solve their medical problems without having to subject themselves to the regime of 'moral entrepreneurs' (Freidson's term) such as lineage elders and priest-healers. In that sense, they are 'liberating' and become important vehicles of individualization (Whyte 1988).[4]

Lack of medical control

What has been called 'liberating' from the patients' point of view is regarded as 'lack of professional control' by medical people. What constitutes the attraction of pharmaceuticals (people's direct access to them) is a cause of concern to the medical profession. The risks of the wrong use of pharmaceuticals are indeed considerable.

The uncontrolled sale of pharmaceuticals in the informal sector is widespread. Many developing countries have a large informal circulation of drugs through pharmacies, stores, markets, itinerant vendors, etc. The medical situation can be described as a self-help culture, partly created by the poor functioning of government services which forces people to 'save themselves' and encourages health workers to privatize their activities in order to increase their income (Van der Geest 1982, 1988). Self-help is also a logical element in the overall process of individualization just presented. This may explain why informal self-medication also occurs in situations where the public system does provide pharmaceuticals: people may prefer not to depend on a doctor or nurse for their medicines.

Cultural processes

Focussing on the actual use of pharmaceuticals, I distinguish three closely related processes which impinge on the way people take their medication: commoditization, cultural reinterpretation and symbolization.

Commoditization

By 'commoditization' I mean that medicines, as 'saleable' items, become part of economic transactions and are thus diverted from the medically controlled distribution channels. Financial constraints as well as affluence affect people's buying and use of pharmaceuticals (cf. Igun 1987).

People with a prescription may not be able to have it filled or decide quite arbitrarily to buy some medicines and leave others. Or they may discover that certain drugs are out of stock and obtain only part of the prescribed medication, not necessarily the 'essential' part (cf. Sangaré & Kessels 1988, Isenalumhe & Oviawe 1988).

Limited income may also make people decide to stop a medication early – when the symptoms abate – to save money. Clients at a market in Cameroon bought very small quantities of drugs because they could not spend more. They rationalized their choice by adapting their opinion about medication to their financial means. A young man suffering from gonorrhoea only bought two tablets of penicillin since he did not have any more money. 'Two is better than none,' he explained (Van der Geest 1991). Whyte (1991) observed a similar phenomenon in Uganda. Customers put their cash on the counter and described the complaint for which they needed drugs: 'Do you have tablets to stop diarrhoea? I want 60 shilling worth' or 'I want white capsules [chloramphenicol]. I have 80 shillings.'

The precarious financial situation in which many people find themselves can be a reason to avoid the formal services and resort to self-medication through the informal sector. Moore et al. (1985) observed that tendency in church-related hospitals in Kenya which had become too expensive for a part of the population. Poor patients stopped visiting the hospital and had to look for cheaper alternatives. A report by the Red Cross (1985) in Uganda writes that almost one-third of the people in rural areas go without any treatment when they are out of money.

In yet another way economic hardship is connected with the use of drugs. Particularly in hectic urban environments, such as Manila, Bombay or Bangkok, many people cannot afford the luxury of being sick or staying away from work to look after a sick child. In that situation people are inclined to symptom-oriented medication to keep going. An overuse of analgesics is the most likely result. Such people are also reluctant to use herbal medicines because they take too much time to prepare and are not strong enough.

Commoditization also works for those who are well to do. Medicines are often considered prestigious items, and people may buy and use them to mark their social status (cf. Tan 1997). I shall discuss this role of pharmaceuticals later on, under the heading of 'symbolisation'.

Cultural reinterpretation

Pharmaceuticals also undergo a process of 'cultural reinterpretation': they move from one context of meaning to another. Produced within a biomedical framework, they are recast into another knowledge system and applied in a way which may be very different from that envisioned by the manufacturer. A well-known example is that local concepts of 'hot' and 'cold' are ascribed as qualities to Western pharmaceuticals. Bledsoe & Goubaud (1985) mention this reasoning in their study among the Mende of Sierra Leone. The same authors found that people paid attention to colour in their selection of medicines. One woman used a yellow anthelmintic drug for malaria '... because she said, when you have malaria your urine is very yellow.' She believed she could expel the sickness with a yellow tablet by 'fighting fire with fire'. Illness and healing are often linked to colour symbolism. Ngubane (1977: 113), in her study of Zulu conceptions of medicine, writes:

> Both black and red are used to expel from the body system what is bad and also to strengthen the body against future attacks. Ridding the body of what is bad and undesirable does not mean that a person is in good health. To regain good health white medicines are used.

The local medical perspective implies a preferential sequence of colours in medication. Red, which stands for transformation, comes first; black and white, which represent static conditions, follow. That sequence may also be preferred in the use of Western pharmaceuticals (see also Fabricant & Hirschhorn 1987).

People in Ghana relate many of their medical complaints to the bowels. Dirt should leave the body as quickly as possible. When it stays too long in the bowels, it starts to produce heat and affects the whole body. Their use of drugs often reflects that concern about dirt. People tend to be focused on cleaning the bowels and reducing excessive heat. Laxatives are very popular and – according to biomedical standards – overused. Analgesics are used as prevention against fever (heat). People take them early in the morning before going to work (Agyepon & Wondergem 1991, Senah 1996).

Etkin et al. (1991) noticed that the Hausa people in Northern Nigeria view illness as a process. A central feature of the theory that guides their selection of medicines is '... the understanding that symptoms of a disease – or even different diseases – develop sequentially, one eventuating from another' (p. 921). They therefore use different medicines at different stages of the disease. Each medicine has specific qualities to fight the symptoms at that particular stage. The authors point out that this idea is now – very rationally – being applied in the use of Western pharmaceuticals. They are used in combination with herbal drugs and their use is stopped as soon as the target symptom has disappeared. The authors give a few examples (e.g. measles) in which Western pharmaceuticals are used according to traditional principles, entirely different from the biomedical ones.

A spectacular example of cultural reinterpretation is found in the use of injections, as we have seen before. Blood takes a central position in illness explanations in many African societies. The injection, which is believed to go directly into the bloodstream, is therefore seen as a highly effective way of curing almost any type of illness. Drips, which work the same way, are increasingly being used to maintain good health (Birungi 1994, Senah 1994).

Basing ourselves upon a large number of case studies, we can safely conclude that very often the actual use of pharmaceuticals by patients – and patients-to-be in the case of preventive medication – diverges widely from biomedical rationality.

Symbolization

Lévi-Strauss (1972) in his famous article has argued that symbols are effective. They *work*. Thus, their concreteness makes pharmaceuticals attractive symbols by which people express emotions as concern, anxiety and love. Doctors show their dedication (or, interestingly, lack of dedication) to patients by giving them medicines. People do the same to their children. Reeler (1996) and Nichter (1989) write that Asian migrants receive medicines from home even though they can be obtained in the place where they are working. Pharmaceuticals are indeed popular gifts. In Uganda a medical assistant of a private clinic told Whyte (1991) that

> ... at least 50% of his customers are people coming on behalf of someone else. Often men come to get medicines for their wives. Men have the money, and they want to show their wives that they care for them...

In certain societies where women are restricted in their movements, men may always buy their wives' medicines (cf. Rasmussen et al. 1996). In Ghana, fathers often give medicine as a gift when a child is born. A favourite medicine for that occasion is *Milk of magnesia*, a laxative (Van der Geest & Whyte 1989: 351). Senah (1994) writes in his study of medicine use in a Ghanaian coastal village:

> Oblefo [a woman] showed me her medicine kit. She explained that in the village, before a woman delivered, it is customary for a 'good' husband to buy certain things including pharmaceuticals as part of the preparations to welcome the expected baby. When I inspected the kit, I found bottles of cod liver oil, cough mixture, *Grycline, Abidec, Gripe Water, Milk of Magnesia* and *Castor* oil... some of the drugs were routinely administered to the child even when there was no need – some have been transformed into prophylaxes.

Like food and like the body, medicines are good to think with and to feel with. They facilitate human relations and mark people's identity. Medicines thus share the role of all commodities: they are not simply consumed; they are symbols of communication and social interaction (cf. Nichter & Vuckovic 1994, Sachs 1989).

The vast literature on the placebo effect tells a similar story. Thanks to their symbolic capacity pharmaceuticals are more effective than can be explained on the basis of their chemical constituents. They are reassuring, they produce confidence, security and hope, the best ingredients for restoring and maintaining health.

Pharmaceuticals are ritual objects. They take a central place in private healing 'ceremonies'. Rituals, stereotypical practices which are carried out in the face of insecurity, help people to pass from one situation to another, from anxiety to tranquillity, from sickness to health, from insomnia to sleep (cf. Haafkens 1997, Uddenberg 1990).

Conclusions

North/South

My focus has been on drug use in developing countries. I have described conditions and processes which not only pose obstacles to the biomedically correct use of drugs but which also obstruct effective research and evaluation of drug use. The informal – and illegal – character of drug use makes a proper assessment of the phenomenon exceedingly painstaking. The little research that has been conducted, however, gives ample reason for concern. Poverty, poor management and lack of balanced information on appropriate drug use cause serious health problems.

This is not to say, however, that such problems do not exist in the industrialized world. Affluence, too, has its health hazards. It may lead to overconsumption of anything including pharmaceuticals. Self-medication flourishes everywhere, also in the shade of a strict control system of pharmaceuticals. Haafkens' study on long-term benzodiazepine use is a telling example.

Rationality

Rationality is a tricky concept, certainly when it is applied to the use of pharmaceuticals. In anthropology there has been a long 'rationality debate'. The centre of the debate was about how much cultural relativism is permitted in defining rationality. After all, rationality is not the prerequisite of Western discursive thinking. Evans-Pritchard's classic in witchcraft, oracles and magic among the Azande in the south of Sudan convincingly argues that believing in the work of witches and the predictive capacity of oracles can be perfectly rational within the framework of the Azande world view. Having accepted the premise that witches exist (no-one has ever proved their non-existence to them) the Azande think not less logically than physicians in their consulting rooms or scientists in their laboratories.

In a similar vein I argue that using pharmaceuticals on the basis of their colour can be a rational thing to do; it makes sense in the philosophy of those who do so. However, the anthropologist's statement does not necessarily imply that each rationality has equal value or is equally effective.

Recognizing (and respecting) different rationalities does not stop people from having their own preference. Anthropologists, too, are cultural beings who are inclined to stick to customs and beliefs which have proved beneficial and trustworthy to them. 'Anything goes' is not the motto of medical anthropology.

By defending the rationality of different beliefs and practices, the anthropologist prepares the way for intercultural communication and understanding, which eventually may lead to a mutual improvement of reasoning. Intercultural communication offers alternative ways of explaining and solving practical life problems, problems of ill health, for example. Taking other people's reasons seriously leads to looking critically at one's own ideas. In the case of drug use, an open and respectful watch for 'inappropriate' practices prevents a dogmatic use of pharmacological knowledge. Medicines may work 'for the wrong reason', and we should be grateful they do. Blinkers would prevent us from reaping these pleasant surprises.

At the same time, we must watch for the dangers of inappropriate drug use. Pharmaceuticals may be consumed in a way which makes sense from an economic, social or symbolic point of view, yet they can be harmful. Fighting the harms of such inappropriate drug use is most likely to succeed if one comes to terms with the rationality of inappropriateness.

How to improve drug use?

My description of the social and cultural-symbolic context of drug use has made it clear that improving the logistics of drug distribution does not automatically lead to a more appropriate use of drugs (Foster 1991a). Even an effective implementation of the essential drugs list is not in the least a guarantee for the 'rational use' of pharmaceuticals (Bennett 1989, Van der Geest et al. 1990).

The most crucial step towards a more appropriate use of pharmaceuticals is informing consumers about 'correct' medication. However, my description of the drugs situation has made clear that such a step is extremely difficult. Medication practices are embedded in social symbolism and local concepts of illness and medicine. They are hard to change. Financial constraints and related factors add to 'irregular' drug use.

But there is also ground for cautious optimism. Consumers across the world are eager to learn about medicine use. Their self-medication culture is characterised by a continuous search for more information on medicines. Appropriate teaching materials should be developed, and the present enormous variety of drugs should be reduced to a small number of cheap and essential medicines. Then people will be better able to judge which medicines are appropriate and how they should be used. Visual aids for the correct use of the most important drugs could be displayed on posters in pharmacies and drugstores and on drug packages. Research is needed to develop suitable symbols for effective instruction and information (cf. Ngoh & Shepherd 1994).

Information on drug use should be integrated in PHC activities. The credibility of community health workers depends to a large extent on their ability to prescribe and dispense drugs. Those who have the most needed drugs at their disposal will also be in a favourable position to dispense the knowledge which is required for appropriate use.

Even the implementation of the Bamako Initiative and the Structural Adjustment Programme and the privatization of state services may have some positive effect as this will most likely make people more aware of the importance of knowing which medicines they need and when and how they should be taken. The first objective of the Bamako Initiative was to render health care more sustainable by making people contribute to it financially. The programme has caused hardship for the indigent, but it also has turned people into more conscious consumers. The free giving of medicines has always had its drawbacks. It made those who received the drugs uncritical and powerless. As 'beggars' they had little to choose and accepted whatever was given to them. Once they have become buyers of medicines, they may be in a better position to voice their demands and complaints and to force health workers and policy-makers to listen to them. Moreover, paying money for drugs will also lead to paying attention to the quality of drugs which are purchased.

Finally, I would like to stress that the improvement of drug use should not be sought in destroying the informal distribution system or in discouraging self-medication. In the present situation in most developing countries, informal medicine distribution and self-care remain indispensable. Solutions for the problems of incorrect medicine use should be pursued in improving the quality of these two institutions and in changing the supply of medicines on the market. Patients should be made more knowledgeable about correct medication, and health workers,' nurses, pharmacists and unqualified vendors of medicines should be encouraged to improve their sale and prescription practices and concentrate on essential drugs.

Notes

1 I thank Susan Foster and Pieter Streefland for their help and comments.
2 *Alophen*, I found out later, is a laxative.
3 For overviews of drug use studies, see: Hardon et al. 1991 and Van der Geest et al. 1996).
4 But after having been 'liberated' from moral entrepreneurs, people may get addicted to certain medicines and become their 'prisoners': freed from people, bound to pharmaceuticals.
5 The International Network for Rational Drugs Use (INRUD) is particularly active in promoting rational prescribing by doctors (see e.g. Laing 1990).

Literature

Agyepon, I. & P. Wondergem
  1991   *Why malaria still prevails: Ethnomedical perceptions of malaria and use of pharmaceuticals in Ghanaian rural communities*. Conference paper, Zeist, The Netherlands.
Alland Jr, A.
  1970   *Adaptation in cultural evolution. An approach to medical anthropology*. New York: Columbia University Press.
Bennett, F.J.
  1989   'The dilemma of essential drugs in Primary Health Care.' *Social Science & Medicine* 28(10): 1085-90.
Birungi, H.
  1994   'Injections as household utilities: Injection practices in Bugosa, Eastern Uganda.' In: N.L. Etkin & M.L. Tan (eds), *Medicines: meanings and contexts*. Quezon City: HAIN, pp. 125-136.
Bledsoe, C.H. & M.F. Goubaud
  1985   'The reinterpretation of Western pharmaceuticals among the Mende of Sierra Leone.' *Social Science & Medicine* 21(3): 275-282.
Bleek, W.
  1978   'Induced abortion in a Ghanaian family.' *African Studies Review* 21: 103-20.
Bloem, M. & I. Wolffers (eds)
  1993   *The Impact of injections on daily medical practice*. Amsterdam: Free University Press.
Chetley, A.
  1989   *Peddling placebos: An analysis of cough and cold remedies*. Amsterdam: Health Action International.

1990   *A healthy business? World health and the pharmaceutical industry.* London: Zed Books.

Etkin, N.L., P.J. Ross & I. Muazzamu
1990   'The indigenization of pharmaceuticals: Therapeutic transitions in rural Hausaland.' *Social Science & Medicine* 30(8): 919-928.

Etkin, N.L. & M.L. Tan (eds)
1994   *Medicines: Meanings and contexts.* Quezon City: HAIN.

Evaluation
1989   *An evaluation of WHO's Action Programme on Essential Drugs.* Unpublished report, Amsterdam: KIT & London: LSHTM.

Fabricant, S.J. & N. Hirschhorn
1987   'Deranged distribution, perverse prescription, unprotected use: The irrationality of pharmaceuticals in the developing world.' *Health Policy & Planning* 2(3): 204-13.

Foster, S.D.
1991a   'Supply and use of essential drugs in Sub-Saharan Africa: Some issues and possible solutions.' *Social Science & Medicine* 32(11): 1201-18.
1991b   'The distribution and use of antimalarial drugs: Not a pretty picture.' In: G.A.T. Targett (ed), *Malaria: waiting for the vaccin.* Chichester: Wiley, pp. 123-128.
1995   'Treatment of malaria outside the formal health services.' *Journal of Tropical Medicine and Hygiene* 98: 29-34.

Haafkens, J.
1997   *Rituals of silence: Long-term tranquilizer use by women in the Netherlands. A social case study.* Amsterdam: Het Spinhuis.

Hardon, A.
1987   'The use of modern pharmaceuticals in a Filipino village: Doctors' prescription and self-medication.' *Social Science & Medicine* 25(3): 277-292.
1990   *Confronting ill health: Medicines, self-care and the poor in Manila.* Quezon City: HAIN.

Hardon, A. et al.
1991   *The provision and use of drugs in developing countries. A review of studies and annotated bibliography.* Amsterdam: Het Spinhuis/HAI.

Igun, U.A.
1987   'Why we seek treatment here: Retail pharmacy and clinical practice in Maiduguri, Nigeria.' *Social Science & Medicine* 24(8): 689-95.

Isenalumhe, A.E. & O. Oviawe
1988   'Polypharmacy: its cost burden and barrier to medical care in a drug-oriented health care system.' *International Journal of Health Services* 18(2): 335-342.

Kanji, N., A., Hardon, J.W., Harnmeijer, M., Mamdani & G. Walt
1992   *Drugs policy in developing countries.* London: Zed Books.

Kanji, N. & A. Hardon
1992   'What has been achieved and where are we now?' In: N. Kanji, A. Hardon, J.W. Harnmeijer, M. Mamdani & G. Walt, *Drugs policy in developing countries.* London: Zed Books, pp. 91-109.
Laing, R.
1990   'Rational drug use: an unsolved problem.' *Tropical Doctor* 20: 101-103.
Lévi-Strauss, C.
1972   'The effectiveness of symbols.' In: C. Lévi-Strauss, *Structural anthropology.* Harmondsworth: Penguin Books, pp. 186-205.
Melrose, D.
1982   *Bitter pills: Medicines and the Third World poor.* Oxford: Oxfam.
Moore, G. et al.
1985   WHO *mission to the joint church medical service of Kenya.* Report of the Catholic Medical Department, Kenya.
Ngoh, L.N. & M.D. Shepherd
1994   'The effect of visual aids and advanced organizers on improving the use of antibiotics in rural Cameroon.' In: N.L. Etkin & M.L. Tan (eds), *Medicines: Meanings and contexts.* Quezon City: HAIN, pp. 227-242.
Ngubane, H.
1977   *Body and mind in Zulu medicine. An ethnography of health and disease in Nyuswa-Zulu thought and practice.* London: Academic Press.
Nichter, M.
1989   *Anthropology and international health: South Asian case studies.* Dordrecht: Kluwer.
Nichter, M. & N. Vuckovic
1994   'Agenda for an anthropology of pharmaceutical practice.' *Social Science & Medicine* 39(11): 1509-1525.
Odoi Adome, R., S.R. Whyte & A. Hardon
1996   *Popular pills: Community drug use in Uganda.* Amsterdam: Het Spinhuis.
Rasmussen, Z.A., M. Rahim, P. Streefland & A. Hardon
1996   *Enhancing appropriate medicine use in the Karakoram Mountains.* Amsterdam: Het Spinhuis.
Red Cross
1985   *Essential drugs management programme. Baseline survey for public education.* Report, Uganda Red Cross Society.
Reeler, A.V.
1990   'Injections: a fatal attraction?' *Social Science & Medicine* 31(10): 1119-1125.
1996   *Money and friendship: Modes of empowerment in Thai health care.* Amsterdam: Het Spinhuis.
Sachs, L.
1989   'Misunderstanding as therapy: Doctors, patients and medicines in a rural clinic in Sri Lanka.' *Culture, Medicine & Psychiatry* 13: 335-349.

Sangaré, M. & P. Kessels

1988   *Rapport d'une recherche exploratoire sur la prescription, l'achat, et l'utilisation des médicaments dans le Cercle de Niono.* Unpublished report.

Senah, K.A.

1994   'Blofa tshofa: Local perception of medicines in a Ghanaian coastal community.' In: N.L. Etkin & M.L. Tan (eds), *Medicines: Meanings and contexts.* Quezon City: HAIN. pp. 83-101.

1997   '*Money be man.' The popularity of medicines in a rural Ghanaian community.* Amsterdam: Het Spinhuis.

Silverman, M. et al.

1982   *Prescriptions for death: The drugging of the Third World.* Berkeley: University of California Press.

Tan, M.L.

1989   *Dying for drugs: Pill power and politics in the Philippines.* Quezon City: HAIN.

1998   '*Magalin na gamot.' Pharmaceuticals and the construction of knowledge and power in the Philippines.* Amsterdam: Het Spinhuis.

Uddenberg, N.

1990   'Medicines as cultural phenomenon.' *Journal of Social and Administrative Pharmacy* 7(4): 179-183.

Van der Geest, S.

1982   'The efficiency of inefficiency: Medicine distribution in South Cameroon.' *Social Science & Medicine* 16(24): 2145-2163.

1987   'Self-care and the informal sale of drugs in South Cameroon.' *Social Science & Medicine* 25(3): 293-305.

1988   'The articulation of formal and informal medicine distribution in South Cameroon.' In: S. van der Geest & S.R. Whyte (eds), *The context of medicines in developing countries: Studies in pharmaceutical anthropology.* Dordrecht: Kluwer, pp. 131-148.

1991   'Marketplace conversations in Cameroon: How and why popular medical knowledge comes into being.' *Culture, Medicine & Psychiatry* 15(1): 69-90.

Van der Geest, S. & A. Hardon

1990   'Self-medication in developing countries.' *Journal of Social and Administrative Pharmacy* 7(4): 199-204.

Van der Geest, S., A. Hardon & S.R. Whyte

1990   'Planning for essential drugs: Are we missing the cultural dimension?.' *Health Policy & Planning* 5(2): 182-185.

Van der Geest, S. & S.R. Whyte

1989   'The charm of medicines: Metaphors and metonyms.' *Medical Anthropology Quarterly* 3(4): 345-367.

Van der Geest, S., S.R. Whyte & A. Hardon
  1996   'The anthropology of pharmaceuticals: A biographical approach.' *Annual Review of Anthropology* 25: 153-178.
Whyte, S.R.
  1988   'The power of medicines in East Africa.' In: S. van der Geest & S.R. Whyte (eds), *The context of medicines in developing countries: Studies in pharmaceutical anthropology*. Dordrecht: Kluwer, pp. 217-234.
  1992   'Pharmaceuticals as folk medicine: Transformations in the social relations of health care in Uganda.' *Culture, Medicine & Psychiatry* 16(2): 163-186.
Wyatt, H.V.
  1984   'The popularity of injections in the Third World: Origins and consequences for poliomyelitis.' *Social Science & Medicine* 19(9): 911-915.

CHAPTER XI

Pharmacological Treasures of the South

Henk van Wilgenburg

Man's first medical treatment was the use of herbs to enhance health. The innate instinct of humans to guard against illness and its consequences led them to empirical health care long before Hippocrates. Today, modern medicine has been tried and tested, but this does not mean that it has displaced herbal medicine. Many rural people and urban poor, especially in Africa, rely on the use of medicinal plants when they are ill. In fact, in many parts of Africa traditional medicine, of which herbal medicine is a vital component, is the major and in some cases the only source of health care available. In several Asian countries traditional medicine is officially recognized. China, for example, is able to provide adequate and constantly improving health care coverage for its vast urban and rural population precisely because it harnesses the precious legacy of traditional medicine (Aregbeyen 1996; Bodeker 1994). In the industrialised world herbal medicine does not have a formal position, but there also herbs play an important role, as 25% of all prescriptions contain materials from higher plants (Seeters 1995).

In 1976 the World Health Organization officially acknowledged the importance of traditional medicine. Two years later, at the conference in Alma Ata, it was proposed that traditional medicine should be included in Primary Health Care. Resolutions in support of national traditional medicine programmes have been adopted by the World Health Assembly, for example, the 1989 resolution drawing attention to herbal medicines as being of great importance to the health of individuals and communities (WHA 42.43).

According to the WHO, as much as 80% of the world's people depend on traditional medicine for their health care needs. The past decade has seen a significant increase in the use of herbal medicines. The results of a preliminary study done on behalf of the WHO has shown that the number of individuals using medicinal plants is large and on the increase, even among young people (IUCN/WHO/WWF 1993).

The natural vegetation of the world, however, is disappearing or being altered at an alarming rate. Many people who live close to nature, depending on its products for their needs, are involved in rapid cultural, social and economic change. These people had a deep understanding of the properties of their local plants – a knowledge that is itself endangered. WHO's strategy 'Health for All by the Year 2000' has made, therefore, conservation of medical plants into an important issue. The 41st World Health Assembly (1988) in its resolution WHA 41.19 drew attention to the 'Chiang Mai Declaration' (Box 1) and endorsed the call for international cooperation and co-ordination to establish a basis for the conservation of medicinal plants, so as to ensure that adequate quantities are available for future generations. This placed medicinal plants, their rational and sustainable use, and their conservation firmly in the arena of public health policy and concern.

Box 1
The Chiang Mai Declaration

Saving lives by saving plants

We, the health professionals and the plant conservation specialists, who have come together for the first time at the WHO/IUCN/WWF International Consultation on Conservation of Medical Plants, held in Chiang Mai, 21-26 March 1988, do hereby reaffirm our commitment to the collective goal of 'Health for All by the Year 2000' through the primary health care approach and to the principles of conservation and sustainable development outlined in the World Conservation Strategy.

We:

- Recognise that medicinal plants are essential in primary health care, both in self-medication and in national health services;
- Are alarmed at the consequences of loss of plant diversity around the world;
- View with grave concern the fact that many of the plants that provide traditional and modern drugs are treated;
- Draw the attention of the United Nations, its agencies and member states, other international agencies and their members and non-governmental organisations to:
  - The vital importance of medicinal plants in health care;
  - The increasing and unacceptable loss of these medicinal plants due to habitat destruction and unsustainable harvesting practises;

- The fact that plant resources in one country are often of critical importance to other countries;
- The significant economic value of the medicinal plants used today and the great potential of the plant kingdom to provide new drugs;
- The continuing disruption and loss of indigenous cultures, which often hold the key to finding new medicinal plants that may benefit the global community;
- The urgent need for international cooperation and coordination to establish programmes for conservation of medicinal plants to ensure that adequate quantities are available for future generations.
- We, the members of the Chiang Mai International Consultation, hereby call on all people to commit themselves to Save Plants that Save Lives.

Chiang Mai, Thailand, 26 March 1988

What are these treasures of the South

Up to about 10% of the dry mass of some plants is made up of chemicals designed for defense. The defense chemicals interact harmfully with the biochemical apparatus of predators and protect plants against infectious diseases caused by viruses, fungi, microbes and other organisms (Abelson 1990).

About 25,000 of these so-called secondary plant constituents have been identified to play an interactive role between the plants and the animal world (Van Genderen, Schoonhoven & Fuchs 1996). It is not surprising, therefore, that quite a number of these constituents can also affect man's physiological processes, such as the functioning of our nervous system (e.g. morphine) or heart (digitalis). Moreover, if these constituents protect plants against viruses, microbes, fungi and parasites, it might well be that these chemicals do the same when we are infected. It is beyond question that plants contain pharmacologically active compounds.

Worldwide, there are 250,000 to 300,000 species of higher plants and ferns. A large fraction of these plants grows in the tropics, especially in the rainforests. Among all the different cultures, more than 10% of these plant species have been used for medical purposes. Less than 0.5% have been studied exhaustively. No more than 120 species have been incorporated into modern medicine, the majority of which came to the attention of pharmaceutical companies because of their use in traditional medical practice. Although most plants grow in tropical zones, fewer than 40 of the 120 species are of tropical origin (Cox & Balick 1994). In the future we can expect that many species of the South will be the source for new medicines (see Box 2).

Box 2

Some of the drugs which were discovered from ethnobotanical leads

- Aspirin, from *Filipendula ulmaria*, reduces pain and inflammation.
- Codeine, from *Papaver somniferum*, eases pain; suppresses coughing.
- Ipecac, from *Psychotria ipecacuanha*, induces vomiting.
- Pilocarpine, from *Pilocarpus jaborandi*, prescribed for glaucoma and dry-mouth syndrome.
- Steroids, from *Dioscorea* species (yam), used to produce cortisone and contraception steroids.
- Colchicine, from *Colchium autimnale* (meadow saffron), used to treat a form of leukaemia.
- Digitalis from *Digitalis purpurea* (foxglove), improves cardiac output.
- Reserpine from the climbing shrub *Rauwolfia serpentina* (Indian snakeroot), lowers blood pressure.
- Vinblastine and vincristine, from *Catharanthus roseus*, since the 1960s prescribed for paediatric leukaemia and Hodgkin's disease.
- Pseudoephedrine, from *Ephedra sinica*, reduces nasal congestion.
- Quinine, from *Cinchona pubescens*, combats malaria.
- Scopolamine, from *Datura stramonium*, eases motion sickness.
- Theophylline, from *Camellia sinensis*, opens bronchial passage.

Plants as a source for (new) medicines

One of the first phytochemists who isolated organic acids was Carl Wilhelm Scheele, a Swede who lived from 1742 till 1786. He studied their salts and made esters from them. After the organic acids the organic alkaloids were discovered in the beginning of the 19th century: Serftüner (1811) found morphine as one of the active principles in opium. Pelletier and Caventou (1820) isolated quinine from *Cortex Cinchonae*. In the 19th century many active compounds from plants were identified and isolated (e.g. quinine, morphine and salicin, better known as the synthesized acetylsalicylic acid or aspirin). Since the discovery of the anticancer drugs vinblastine and vincristine in the 1950s, however, few main discoveries of plant-derived drugs have been made. Until a decade ago the pharmaceutical industry was not seriously interested in medicinal plants as a source of medicines. Cultures of fungi (for antibiotics) and synthetic pharmaceuticals were considered to be more important. Moreover, advances in synthetic chemistry and molecular biology promised to supply new means for designing drugs in the laboratories of the Pharma-industry.

Natural products, however, offer a rich source for new chemical structures. For example, in 1985 a total of 3500 new chemical structures were discovered, and some 2619 of them were isolated from higher plants (Abelson, 1990). Fast and (semi-)automatic screening methods have been developed now, based on molecular methods, that can perform between 50,000 to 150,000 tests for specific biological activity per week (Zeelen 1997). Due to these advanced screening methods and also new techniques for revealing the chemical structure of the constituents, such as chromatography, mass spectrometry and nuclear magnetic resonance (NMR), the industry has shown a renewed interest in plant compounds.

The story of antimalarials parallels that of other pharmaceuticals

The historical development of antimalarials shows a typical pattern of alternation of emphasis on natural resources and synthetic sources, with technological development as a crucial variable. Evidently, sociopolitical factors as well as other malaria control strategies including the production of vaccines, the use of insecticides, the promotion of impregnated bednets and the sanitary approach also shape the demand for antimalarials. Pelletier and Caventou (1820) isolated quinine from the bark of *Cinchona* trees. The drug became popular in colonial days, but particularly during the two World Wars it was no longer possible to keep up the supply. Between 1930 and 1960 many synthetic antimalarial drugs were developed, the most notable of them being chloroquine (and amodiaquine and pyrimethamine). In 1947, over 600 plants of 126 families were screened against *Plasmodium gallinaceum* in chicks and other *Plasmodium* species in ducks. Due to the difference in the nature of avian and human malaria parasites, it remained an open question of whether these results could be transferred to human malaria parasites. Unfortunately, during the early 1970s *P. falciparum* malaria parasites were found to be developing resistance against most of the quinoline-based drugs. In recent years about 250,000 compounds have been synthesized and tested for their antimalarial potency. Only one of them, mefloquine, has been developed into an antimalarial drug at a cost of USD 150 million.

As a result of the poor outcome with synthetic compounds, researchers have focussed more attention during the last 15 years on plants as sources of alternative antimalarial drugs. Most of the plants being investigated are those which have been used for centuries as antimalarials or those which belong to families or genera with proven antimalarial properties.

An efficient and semi-automated method to screen for drug inhibition of *Plasmodium falciparum* growth *in vitro* was developed at the end of the 1970s and facilitates the research. The *in vitro* antimalarial screening procedure against *P. falciparum* is based on the ability of drugs to inhibit uptake of the radiolabelled nucleic acid precursor [3H]-hypoxanthine by the malaria parasite.

Especially the isolation of artemisinine from *Artemisia annua* (Chinese antimalarial herb) has rekindled efforts to search for antimalarials from medicinal plants. Based also on earlier studies, a number of plant families (Amaryllidaceae, Annonaceae, Meliaceae, Menispermaceae, Rubiaceae, Rutaceae and Simaroubaceae) known to contain antimalarial constituents have been investigated. Various classes of chemical structures have been isolated (see Box 3), such as alkaloids, limonoids, quassinoids, terpenoids and dihydrochalcones (Nkunya 1992).

Box 3
Chemical structures isolated from plants
in the search for antimalarials

Alkaloids

The first known was quinine from the barks of the *Cinchona* tree (1820) from Latin America.

Febrifugine (from *Dichora febrifuga*, Chinese antimalarial plant) was isolated in the 1980s, but is reported to lead to liver toxicity in humans. Tetrandrine (isolated from *Stephania tetranda*, used in China for antirheumatic and analgetic properties and related to alkaloids from *Trisclisia* species, used in Ghana as antimalarials) potentiates the effectiveness of other antimalarial drugs, such as chloroquine (40-fold) and also artemisine, against multidrug-resistant malarial cells, without blocking Ca^{2+} channels.

Another 40 alkaloids have been isolated and tested *in vitro* and *in vivo* (in mice), some being less active than chloroquine, or showing toxic effects in therapeutic doses. Vinblastine is one of them, which inhibits the growth of the trophozoite stage of the parasite.

Limonoids

Of these compounds isolated from members of the families Meliaceae, Rutaceae and Cneoraceae, all used for medicinal purposes, 5 showed a mild antimalarial activity.

Quassinoids

More than 30 have been isolated from the family Simaroubaceae and are known to be antineoplastic in vivo. In traditional medicine these plants are used for the treatment of cancer, amoebic dysentery, malaria and other ailments. Their antimalarial activity parallels their antileukaemic activity. Some of these compounds are very promising as antimalarial drugs.

Terpenoids

The most potent antimalarial terpenoid known so far is artemisine, first isolated in 1972 from the Chinese antimalarial plant *Artemisia annua*. Another 20 terpenoids are under investigation. Also, the antitumour drug taxol (from *Taxus brevifolia*) has been found to be active against *P. falciparum*.

Other compounds

Another 30 compounds belonging to different chemical classes and crude extracts, e.g. 57 Tanzanian medicinal plants, including nine *Uvaria* species, have been shown to have antimalarial properties.

Investigations of medicinal plants are now giving leads about potent and non-toxic antimalarial drugs. Whether these new antimalarials will, in time, become available and will be of any benefit for the people in the South remains to be seen. It is well established that intake of appropriate doses of some malaria drugs at specified time intervals (e.g. fortnightly) can provide effective protection against malaria. Hence it can be correctly argued that people resident in regions with endemic malaria should be encouraged to take such prophylactic doses of malaria drugs in order to manage and eventually control the disease. Unfortunately, for various reasons, including poverty, poor health service delivery and cultural notions emphasizing cure instead of prevention, prophylaxis cannot be maintained by people in regions endemic to malaria (Van der Geest, this volume).

Search for anti-cancer drugs

Although in general the Pharma-industry did not show much interest in plants from 1950-1980, the National Cancer Institute (NCI) in the USA formed an exception. NCI screened chemicals from 35,000 plants, collected at random from all parts of the world, during the period 1952-1982, with the aim to find new anticancer drugs (Nicolaou, Rodney & Potier 1996). Some of the extracts were effective, but with harmful side effects. In 1967 a chemical component, taxane, was isolated from a tree called *Taxus brefolia*, the Pacific yew, known by native American tribes who used the bark as a disinfectant and a treatment for skin cancer. The compound was named taxol. Initially, the NCI did not consider the compound particularly promising. Other drugs worked just as well or better than taxol. But between 1978 and 1988 researchers discovered some unique properties of taxol in attacking cancer cells, particularly with regard to the binding to microtubules and inhibition of mitosis. In 1991 taxol made headlines as a breakthrough treatment of ovarial cancer. Women suffering from advanced ovarian cancer who took taxol in combination with another anticancer medication lived on average 14 months longer.

But there was a problem: taxol had to be extracted from the bark of a slowly growing tree. A 100-year-old tree provides only one gram of taxol, i.e. half the amount needed for one treatment. Harvesting the trees would cause irreparable harm to the ecosystem, and supplies would last only five years. Chemists, however, exhibited a serious interest in taxol. With 112 atoms taxol is aesthetically and scientifically appealing. Synthesis turned out to be possible but extremely difficult. In 1994 scientists at the National Center of Scientific Research in France succeeded in making taxol and taxotere by semisynthesis, starting with the leaves of the common European yew *Taxus baccata*. Mankind won a new pharmaceutical against cancer.

What can be learned from this case? A random search for new leads is time-consuming and expensive: a single success, the discovery of taxol, among the screened chemicals from 35,000 plants over a period of 30 years is a poor result. In general, it does take a long time, on average 10 years, to develop a new medicine. The cost of developing a drug is high: between USD 100-300 million. Although taxol and taxatere are of herbal origin, their price on the market will be high and not affordable for the poor. The natural resources are often limited. The traditional property rights are worth nothing, when these natural resources are exploited for use worldwide. The plant itself is no longer available to the local people for use as a traditional herbal medicine.

Renewed interest for natural resources

Today, the NCI and the Pharma-industry employ several plant-gathering strategies. No longer are plants sampled only at random. Other approaches in use are:

Phylogenetic surveys: investigation of close relatives of plants known to produce useful compounds. For example. *Artemisia annua*, known as a traditional Chinese medicine, was described for its antimalarial properties as early as 350 AD. Artemisine was isolated in 1972 as the most potent compound. *Artemisia annua* belongs to the genus *Artemisia*, a group consisting of 180 species. Many of these species are used by country people in different cultures for intermittent fever and also contain useful compounds.

The ecological approach: studying the interaction between organisms. Plants use secondary plant constituents for defense. The way plants interact with predators, viruses, fungi and microbes can reveal their special healing properties.

The ethnobotanical approach: finding new leads by investigating the use of plants in traditional medicine (see Box 4). It was found, for example, that 86% of the plants used by Samoan healers display significant biological activity.

Box 4
How ethnobotanists work

Ethnobotanists work as follows:

Collection: 1 kg /species with permission of the healers, village chiefs, landowners and governments and 4-5 samples of a plant to serve as 'voucher'.

Dry plants or alcohol extracts are stored for transport. In the laboratory molecules are extracted by immersing them in various solvents. Potential drugs are screened on bioassays – usually automated.

If an assay is positive, another 50-100 kg is needed to isolate the molecule and to determine its structure. If possible a synthetic version will be made for further investigation. If the test molecule has a significant activity – also known as a lead compound – evaluation proceeds. Pharmacological, toxicological tests and clinical trials are performed, and finally the new compound can be registered as a regular medicine.

How many new leads have been identified by these approaches since the 1980s is unknown. Pharmaceutical producers keep this a secret in the stages of development before the final registration. Two drug candidates discovered in this way have reached clinical trials and are being developed by Shaman Pharmaceuticals (California). The active components come from a plant that grows in Latin America. One formulation shows activity against respiratory viruses, while the second may be administered for treating infections caused by the herpes simplex virus. Some other leads are promising: as an anti-inflammatory drug, for gastrointestinal disorders, and as an antihelmintic. Prostratin from the tree *Homalanthus nutans* (Samoa, Polynesia, used against yellow fever) shows potential anti-HIV activity.

Can ethnobotany help local communities adapt to changing circumstances?

Ethnobotanical practices have been modified to ensure safeguarding of the rights of people in the South to their indigenous knowledge, which implies that they benefit from any commercial discoveries based on their knowledge (Koerts 1995). The International Cooperative Biodiversity Groups (ICBG) programme comprises, for example, grants to drug discovery groups prospecting in Latin America and Africa, requiring such groups to pursue three goals: drug discovery, conservation of the environment and genetic resources of the source country, and development of sustainable economic activities for the local people (Rouhi 1997). In Surinam, the ICBG works with indigenous forest people living in the interior of the country. The Surinam group is particularly strong and effective in its conservation and economic development efforts because of its partnership with Conservation International, based in Washington. In Costa Rica another group, the biodiversity institute INBio, established a collaboration with the pharmaceutical giant Merck. The initial agreement provided Merck with a limited number of plant, insect, fungal and environmental samples from Costa Rica's protected areas for study. In return INBio receives research funding from Merck: about USD 1 million for 1997 and 1998 combined. Shaman Pharmaceuticals founded 'Healing Forest Conservancy', a non-profit organisation that aims at conservation of biodiversity and promised that a certain percentage of the gains will be earmarked for this organisation. Stocks of Shaman Pharmaceuticals are promoted as 'politically correct'. Dutch companies are also aware of their responsibilities in protecting the properties of local communities. Thanks to financial assistance from Biohorma, the licensed agency for the Benelux producing and supplying natural remedies, and from one of the largest energy companies in the Netherlands, a project was initiated by the University of Utrecht in 1994 which has set aside a 2400 hectare piece of land in the Amazon rain forest for conservation.

If eventually ethnobotany leads to the development of a new potent drug, the problem of royalty arises. This is demonstrated in the following example: The pharmaceutical giant Eli Lilly produces vinblastine and vincristine extracted from the rosy periwinkle, *Catharanthus roseus*, cultivated in Texas, a plant originally brought from Madagascar. But the USD 180 million business derived from *Catharanthus* is of little benefit to Madagascar. Madagascar claims *Catharanthus* as their property and accuses the pharmaceutical company of having stolen the plant (Oliver & Backhouse 1995).

Although the Pharma-industry can play a role in the protection of the biodiversity and in a lesser extent perhaps also in saving some of the indigenous knowledge of herbal medicine, it is also clear that the people in the South will hardly benefit from the new discoveries as long as companies from the North are involved, as they have the capacity to siphon away the natural raw materials at a very low cost and then sell the processed products, also in the source countries of the original resource, at a very high price.

The benefits which people in the South derive from use of their herbal resources by Northern pharma-industries is also limited because the pharmaceutical industries have a lack of interest in the production of medicines for tropical diseases (see also Terpstra & Smits, this volume). To quote the research director of a company:

> Of course, we could go into a big program on, say, tropical sleeping sickness (or Chagas disease). We might put in three, four, or five million dollars a year. In five or ten years, we might hit on a useful new compound that could help a lot of people in Africa or South America. They would like to have it. They have the disease but not the money. My stockholders would have my scalp (Silverman et al. 1982:99).

The position of herbal medicine in the South

Traditional healing in the South in the course of time has come under pressure from novel cures for infectious diseases that revealed the superiority of 'white man's capsules'. This course of events has greatly affected the prestige of the local healers and has also opened a market for expensive and less necessary Western drugs. Apart from posing a heavy drain on foreign cash reserves, easily available and often equally effective traditional equivalents have been forced into disuse and oblivion.

Studies looking specifically at health-seeking behaviour in relation to malaria and other endemic diseases in developing countries indicate that self-diagnosis is followed by self-medication (Van der Geest, this volume). The first choice involves the over-the-counter (OTC) drugs. However, the wide range, types and formulations of OTC drugs including antimalarials available in the retail outlets constitute a major health hazard. The wide accessibility and use of modern drugs has negative consequences such as irrational use of often inessential, potentially dangerous drugs, development of resistant strains, iatrogenesis and even death.

In the developing world a substantial part of the population has no access to good quality public health services. Due to the effects of processes such as political disintegration and poor economic performance, primary health care and essential medicines are becoming even less easily available than in the past (Chabot et al. 1995; Streefland 1994). Under such conditions other sources of care, including herbal medicine, may gain prominence.

The majority of the people in the South continue to depend heavily on traditional medicine. This is not only because these medicines are easily available and are also relatively cheap, but also because traditional medicine fulfils a unique role in health care. It has its own niche and is seen as complementary to modern health care. Moreover, in peripheral rural areas only traditional healing and herbal self-care may be at hand.

A task for governments in the promotion of herbal medicine production and use

In view of the current crisis in the provision of modern health care, particularly in African countries, there is every justification for governments to promote knowledge and understanding of herbal medicine. Thus, Aregbeyen (1996) recommends that African governments provide health education on herbal remedies and on the identification of medicinal plants and herbs which are used by different communities for the treatment of common diseases.

Besides, if countries of the South could produce their own drugs from their own plants, that will greatly reduce their dependence on the imports of expensive medicine from developed countries. Aregbeyen (1996) mentions in this respect inventorying and documenting medicinal plants and herbs, establishing botanical gardens for their preservation, setting up of a network of laboratories to assess their efficacy, and establishing dosage norms for the most efficacious use of herbal extracts.

Some promising initiatives in African countries, as for example the Centre of Research on Pharmacopoeia and Traditional Medicine (CURPHAMETRA) in Rwanda (see Box 5), have demonstrated that preserving the heritage of medicinal plants and traditional medicine by rationally exploiting these natural resources for their own benefit is feasible.

Box 5
CURPHAMETRA

In 1980 the National University of Rwanda set up CURPHAMETRA as an autonomous and multidisciplinary research centre with a pilot production department to produce medicines from local raw materials, i.e. traditional prescription and medicinal plants. In order to benefit from the information held by the traditional healers a Dispensary (or Community Clinic) of Traditional Medicine was organized, where healers and doctors could carry out consultations with patients.

The advantages of this set up are:
- it validates knowledge that has been handed down from previous generations;
- it reduces imports;
- it creates jobs at several levels;
- it makes appropriate medicines available to the population at a reasonable price;
- it opens up the possibility for export;
- it protects and preserves the natural environment.

The production of medicines started from plants already known and described in pharmacopoeias, since it took less time and did not require long and costly research. New drugs, for example, an antimycotic, have also been developed as a result of information obtained from the healers. The plants were either grown or picked. For the production of different extracts, an extraction and distillation unit was set up. Several medicines produced as syrups, solutions, tablets, ointments and powders were sold wholesale to hospitals, health centres and community clinics or dispensaries and retail to private pharmacies.

They included:
- mouth disinfectant: *Eucalyptus, Mentha*
- anti-cough syrup: *Plantago*
- anti-cough syrup: *Eucalyptus, Datura*

- anti-cough solution: Datura, Thymus, Eucalyptus
- anti-spasmodic syrup: *Datura*
- anti-inflammatory and healing ointment: *Calendula*
- anti-rheumatic solution: *Capsicum*

Unfortunately, due to the unstable political situation in Ruanda, this initiative has come to an end. However, the possibility and the feasibility of processing traditional medicines from own resources in a cheap way acceptable for both healers and doctors has been demonstrated.

Partly due to the encouragement from the WHO, an increasing number of governments and other agencies are fully aware of the importance of medicinal plants in providing primary health care to the people. Many experts and practitioners now have a deep understanding of the issues involved. But without a solid foundation of political commitment, essential research and management programmes may not be completely secure at times of political change or financial stringency.

In accordance with the 'Chiang Mai Declaration' (Box 1), in 1993 the WHO, the International Union for the Conservation of Nature (IUCN) and the World Wildlife Fund (WWF) jointly published the *Guidelines on the Conservation of Medicinal Plants*. Specifically, these guidelines for ethnobotany and ethnopharmacology include:

1 Each country should identify and support one or more institutions to plan, co-ordinate and implement ethnobotanical surveys.
2 The selected institution(s) should implement a nationwide programme of surveys on the use of plants for medicinal purposes in traditional societies.
3 The data on ethnobotany should be catalogued and analysed but only disseminated is such a way that the communities providing the data would receive benefits from any commercial use of the information.
4 The Ministry of Health should incorporate proven traditional remedies into national programmes of Primary Health Care.
5 Traditional Health Practitioners should constitute themselves into national bodies.

These guidelines and recommendations like those given by Aregbeyen (1996) are certainly not exhaustive. Other measures will be necessary, such as preventing the theft of the natural resources by foreign institutions and their middlemen, preservation of indigenous knowledge, keeping up herbaria and botanical gardens, to mention a few. Not only governments, but also NGOs can contribute successfully to these tasks (Wolffers 1990; Le Grand et al. 1993).

In conclusion, I hope that the efforts of national governments and the recommendations from the international organisations will result jointly in initiatives enabling countries in the South to look more inwardly and to use their own treasures, rather than continuing to rely on expensive, imported medicines which have thus far consumed a substantial part of their national finances.

Literature

Abelson. P.H.
> 1990 'Medicine from plants.' *Science* 247: 513.

Aregbeyen, J.B.O.
> 1996 'Traditional herbal medicine for sustainable PHC.' *Indigenous Knowledge and Development Monitor* 4: 14-15.

Bodeker, G.
> 1994 'Traditional health knowledge and public policy.' *Nature and Resources* 30: 5-16.

Chabot, J., J.W. Harnmeijer & P.H. Streefland
> 1995 *African PHC in times of economic turbulence.* Amsterdam: KIT Press.

Cox, P.A. & M.J. Balick
> 1994 'The Ethnobotanical approach to drug discovery.' *Scientific American*, June 1994, pp. 60-65.

IUCN/WHO/WWF
> 1993 *The guidelines on the conservation of medicinal plants.* Somerset: Castle Cary Press.

Koerts, P.J.
> 1995 'Farma-industrie zoekt het geheim van het oerwoud.' *Het Financiële Dagblad*, 7 Febr. 1995.

Le Grand, A., P.H. Streefland & L. Sri-Ngernyuang
> 1993 'Enhancing appropriate drug use: The contribution of herbal drug promotion.' *Social Science & Medicine* 36(8): 1023-1037.

Nicolaou, K.C., K. Guy & P. Potier
> 1996 'Taxoids: New weapons against Cancer.' *Scientific American*, June 1996, pp. 84-88.

Nkunya, M.H.H.
> 1992 'Progress in the search for antimalarials.' *Napreca Monograph Series* No. 4.

Oliver, C.E. & M. Backhouse
  1995   'The role of medicine in conservation and the treat to biodiversity in Madagascar.' *Medical & Global Survival* 4: 243-247.
Rouhi, A.M.
  1997   'Seeking drugs in natural products.' *Chemical & Engineering News* 75: 14-29.
Seters, A.P.
  1995   'A remedial treasure in our tropical timberyard?' *Medical & Global Survival* 2: 248-251.
Silverman, M., P. Lee & M. Lydecker
  1982   *Prescriptions for death: The drugging of the Third World.* Berkeley: University of California Press.
Streefland, P.H.
  1994   'Shaping the context of drug use: Availability of pharmaceuticals at the frontier of cosmopolitan medicine.' In: N.L. Etkin & M.L. Tan (eds), *Medicines: Meanings and contexts.* Quezon City: HAIN, pp. 209-224.
Van Genderen, H., L.M. Schoonhoven & A. Fuchs
  1996   *Chemisch ecologische flora van Nederland en België.* Utrecht: KNNV Uitgeverij.
Wolffers, I.
  1990   *The role of traditional medicine in PHC.* Amsterdam: VU University Press.
World Health Organization
  1978   *Alma-Ata 1978: Primary health care.* Report of the international conference of primary health care. Health for All Series, No. 1.
Zeelen, F.J.
  1997   'Snelle screeningsmethode boeiend perspectief.' *Conceptuur* 13: 6.

Contributors

JARL CHABOT is a public health physician. He supported the governments of Angola and Guinea-Bissau in their efforts to build up their health care system and has also worked extensively in a supportive capacity in the Sahel region. He headed the health care and disease control department at the Royal Ttropical Institute and currently works as a freelance consultant.

HENK VAN WILGENBURG is a biologist and pharmacologist at the Academic Medical Centre's pharmacological laboratory. He coordinates projects aimed at transfering knowledge between Europe, China, East Africa and Surinam. His interests include neuropharmacology and ethnopharmacology.

SJAAK VAN DER GEEST is a cultural anthropologist and professor of medical anthropology at the University of Amsterdam. He has done fieldwork in Ghana and Cameroon. His research interests include the social and cultural context of medicines, the meaning of old age, and ideas and practices concerning fertility.

HENK SMITS is a biologist who previously worked at the University of Amsterdam and is currently employed at the department of biomedical research of the Royal Tropical Institute.

WIEPKO TERPSTRA is a medical doctor and microbiologist. He worked for several years in Surinam and Tanzania. He currently heads the department of biomedical research at the Royal Tropical Institute.

PIET KAGER is an internal diseases specialist and professor of tropical medicine at the University of Amsterdam. He worked in a government hospital in Zaire and in the Medical Research Centre in Kenya.

JANE KUSIN is a medical doctor and professor of tropical nutrition at the University of Amsterdam. Her interests include maternal child health & nutrition and nutrition policy. She conducted research in Benin, Kenya, Indonesia and the Philippines. She also headed the department of nutrition and currently works as a consultant at the Royal Tropical Institute.

PIETER STREEFLAND studied sociology and is professor of applied development sociology at the University of Amsterdam. His interests include the social and cultural context of epidemics, immunization, and the relationship between poverty and health. He did fieldwork in Bangladesh, India, Nepal, and Pakistan. In addition, he headed the primary health care department and is currently a senior research fellow at the Royal Tropical Institute.

ABRAM DE SWAAN is professor of sociology and chairs the Amsterdam School for Social Research at the University of Amsterdam. In *In care of the State* (1988) he wrote about the formation of the welfare state. In 1997/98 he was appointed to the "chaire Européenne" at the Collège de France.

ANITA HARDON is a medical biologist and medical anthropologist and an associate professor at the University of Amsterdam. She did fieldwork in the Philippines. Her research interests include the use of medicines, reproductive health, and the sociocultural aspects of medical technology.

STUART BLUME studied chemistry at Oxford University. From 1977-80 he was Scientific Secretary of the (UK) *Committee on Social Inequalities in Health* (Black Committee). He became a professor of science dynamics at the University of Amsterdam in 1982.

CORLIEN VARKEVISSER is a medical anthropologist with a degree in public health. She conducted research and provided training in support of PHC and infectious disease control (leprosy, TB, HIV/AIDS) in many African countries. At present she coordinates the international course in health development at the Royal Tropical Institute and is professor of interdisciplinary research on health and development at the University of Amsterdam.